By Tara L. McGuire

Copyright c 2014 by Tara L. McGuire. All rights reserved. Published by Tara L. McGuire.

By law this work is protected by copyright and therefore no one is permitted to copy, broadcast, transmit, show or play in public, adapt or change in any way the content of this book for any other purpose whatsoever without prior written permission from Tara L. McGuire.

taramcguire@mac.com

Other books by Tara L. McGuire:

BIRTH UNHINDERED

http://www.birthunhindered.com

****

About the Author

Tara L. McGuire is an activist and author on the topics of health and healing, pregnancy, birth, personal growth and empowerment. She has a history as a Certified Childbirth Educator (CCE) and CCE Trainer through BirthWorks® International, as well as acting as a birth attendant. Currently, Tara is a certified yoga instructor and co-owns and operates Epídavros Center for Wellbeing and Epídavros Yoga Studio with her husband, Don. In addition to these activities, Tara is a home-schooling mother of four children and surrogate mother to one.

Tara's purpose and mission statement:

The purpose of my life is to experience joy and passion by helping myself, and others, live life to its highest potential.

****

Disclaimer

This book is intended to serve as a resource and educational guide. Neither the author nor the publisher is engaged in rendering professional advice or services to the reader. The ideas, procedures, and suggestions in this book are not intended as a substitute for consulting a physician or a licensed health care practitioner, but as an adjunct to such care. The information and opinions expressed here are believed to be accurate, based on the best judgment available to the author. The author shall not be liable or responsible for any loss, injury, or damage allegedly arising from any information or suggestion in this book, nor is the author responsible for the reader's specific health or allergy needs that may require medical supervision or for any adverse reactions to the techniques, procedures, or products discussed in this book. The publisher is not responsible for errors or omissions.

****

Acknowledgements

I would like to thank, first and foremost, God for giving me the tenacity never to settle, but to strive continually for abundance in all things. Secondly, I thank my partner in life and in love, Don. Without him, I never would have the care or ability to heal myself. He is the wind beneath my wings and the reason that I care to fly. I would also like to thank my mother and father for teaching me to believe in myself and that anything is possible with faith. And, last, but not least, my editor and friend, Tomme Fent.

****

Table of Contents

Introduction	p 5

Section One
Let's Get Started	p 9
Causes of Decline	p 9
Down in the Ditch	p 17
Quality of Mind	p 20
Make a Decision	p 25
Path of Healing	p 27
Study	p 29

Section Two
Heal Your Body	p 32
Reduce Stress	p 32
Clear Toxins	p 37
The 5 Organs of Elimination	p 40
Additional Techniques	p 48
The Diet	p 56
Sound Therapy	p 76
Rest and Relaxation	p 79
Exercise	p 80
Alignment	p 84

Section Three
Heal Your Mind	p 86
Power of Thoughts	p 86
Worry	p 87
Self Talk	p 88
Visualization	p 90

Section Four
Heal Your Spirit..p 91
In Closing..p 93
About the Author...p 99

Introduction

I am a yoga instructor and co-owner of a wellness center, and sometimes it seems that my whole adult life has been about trying to be my healthiest. This book is a compilation of twenty-plus years of learning, practicing, and making sense of the body, the mind, the spirit, and the intricate relationship between them. It is a compilation of truths I have found that bring me to a state of vitality, strength, and peace. It is my hope that this book will bring you some of the same, and you will live out your years at a higher level of existence as a result of your endeavors to be well.

It is my firmly held belief that our bodies are miraculous, and if we give them the right elements, put them in the right environment, and bring them into harmony with mind and spirit, they will heal. Nearly every sick person has the ability to feel better. Even if full recovery from your situation isn't possible, you CAN live more fully and feel more vitality. And for many of you, it is completely possible that you can heal yourself!

I've often said, "I'm not gifted with good health," and while this can seem like a pessimist's view, I don't think so. While it's easy to see this statement as negative, I see it as positive. The alternatives would be, "I'm cursed with bad health," or "I'm sick," or "I've got X disease." So, for me, "I'm not gifted with good health" is a positive spin on my very real situation.

My journey through life in this physical body has been interesting, to say the least. In my teens, I had many symptoms of illness, but through the ignorant bliss of youth, I ignored them. Once I was in my 20s, my weak constitution became much more obvious. I was, in that decade, told that I was in the early stages of lupus. In addition to this, I had been treated for and/or diagnosed with secondary infertility, hypothyroidism, goiter, eczema, chronic sinusitis, hypoglycemia, alopecia, acne, bruising easily, depression, constant viral infections, and more.

Then came my 30s, which were filled with a super abundance of stress, bringing on symptoms of stroke and possibly heart attack. (Mind you, I had always stayed right around my ideal weight, exercised, and eaten what most Americans would consider healthy.) These symptoms lingered with me for more than seven years before I finally got a definitive diagnosis.

Now that I am past the 40 year mark, I see things in a new light. A process of study, practice, and understanding is what has set me up to have a bright future. I have been diagnosed with familial spinocerebellar ataxia (most likely gluten ataxia), essential tremor with dystonia (torticollis), gluten intolerance, leaky gut syndrome, and adrenal fatigue. These diagnoses have not dampened my enthusiasm for the future. Because I have been proactive in sorting out what is going on in my body, and in learning how to care for myself, my future is going to be brighter and healthier than the average person's.

- Menopausal symptoms
- Secondary infertility
- Muscle pain
- Joint pain
- Numbness and tingling
- Formication
- Poor balance
- Impaired gait
- Difficulty waking
- Sense of falling
- Clumsiness
- Compromised proprioception
- Difficulty swallowing
- Difficulty speaking
- Hypoglycemia
- Hypothyroidism
- Eczema
- Acne
- Alopecia
- Anemia
- Easy bruising
- Cold hands and feet
- Neuropathy

It is my heartfelt hope that the information, practices, and suggestions presented in this book will encourage you to embark on the exciting journey of learning to relieve your own symptoms, whatever they may be. Heal Yourself!

I may not be gifted with good health, but DAMN if I am earning it for myself!

Through my own self-care and study, I have alleviated and/or eliminated the following symptoms:

- Mood swings
- Stress
- Anxiety
- Depression
- Fatigue
- Poor memory
- Brain fog
- Inability to concentrate
- Adrenal fatigue
- Energy crashes
- Slow wound healing
- Chronic infections
- Headaches
- Sinus infections
- Teeth grinding
- Sleep apnea
- TMJ
- Seasonal allergies
- Frequent colds
- Shortness of breath
- Chest pain
- Heart palpitations/fluttering
- Atrial fibrillation
- Arrhythmia
- Nausea
- Abdominal pain
- Gas and bloating
- Constipation and diarrhea
- PMS

Lets Get Started

Causes of Decline

While some believe the causes of decline in our physical health can be attributed to one thing or another, I actually believe that is not the case. I believe we arrive at a state of disease through a string of bad scenarios. Then there are some who seem not only to have a string of bad scenarios, but ones that line up at the right time to create the "perfect storm." These would be the individuals who lived seemingly healthy lives until they suddenly took a dramatic downturn.

Major contributors to a decline in our health include: stress; toxins – in our environment, our food and water, our toiletries, our medications, and even our thoughts; and lifestyle choices. Let's take a look at the ways each of these can cause stress to the body.

One of the biggest reasons we lose our good health is STRESS. Chronic stress is linked to the six leading causes of death. What makes us sick ultimately moves us closer to death. Our body's reaction to stress is not, inherently, a bad thing; in fact, our bodies react to stress in a way designed to protect us. When we are frightened or threatened in some way, the sympathetic nervous system (SNS) is triggered, kicking the body into "fight or flight" mode. Sadly, the body couldn't care less whether this is a situation of real and imminent danger, or emotional/mental duress. Even if the stressor is only in your mind, your SNS gears up and is ready to party, causing the following to occur:

- You get a burst of energy.
- Non-essential body functions are shut down.
- Digestion is slowed, and your immune system is weakened.
- Heart rate is increased.
- Blood pressure is increased.
- Adrenaline helps pump blood to your major muscles, so you can run or fight.
- Immune system function is slowed, because it is unnecessary during fight or flight.
- Sensitivity to pain is temporarily lowered.

While this situation is helpful if you are being chased by a gunman, or are in the middle of an earthquake, these responses, for the most part, are unnecessary in dealing with day-to-day life. The trick is to learn to change either the situation causing the stress, or the way in which you think about it.

I'm the last person in the world to underestimate stressful situations. I know, all too well, how tough stress can be. There are times when we CAN change a situation to remove stress, and there are times when we can't change the situation and must, instead, change the way we think about it. Here's an example from my own life. My first marriage was a poor match, and made for wrong reasons, but we were both good people who wanted very much to make it work. After 14 difficult years, my husband and I knew that as soon as our four kids left home, we would get divorced. However, we ultimately decided to part ways long before our children were grown. I found myself as a single, home-schooling mom of four children. My unwillingness to put my children in school at that point added another deep level of stress to an already-stressful situation.

Okay, so I identified that a situation was causing me stress, but I didn't feel the situation could be changed. So now what? I had to change the way I thought about it. For now, I'm just presenting the issue – the fact that stress can play a major factor in the decline of good health. We will address tactical ways to manage stress in a future chapter.

If stress is a leader in the decline of good health, what follows it? Our TOXIC world is an easy second. A person doesn't have to search very long to find that we are exposed to environmental toxins continually, and these very toxins are causing a huge assault on our wellbeing. Unless we eat a strictly organic diet, the very act of eating causes us to consume chemicals that cause cancer, dementia, and more. Minimally, they assault our immune system and clog our liver. Often, they attack our nervous system, as well. Then, we pour a glass of water from the tap, and take in over 100 basic contaminants that are common everywhere, plus fluoride, if your district adds it. You filter your drinking water? Great. Do you bathe? Your skin is your largest organ, and five minutes in a hot bath or shower are equivalent to drinking that same water for one month. The Environmental Working Group (EWG), a non-profit, non-partisan organization dedicated to protecting human health and the environment, performed a 2½-year study of more than 22 million tap water quality tests from nearly 40,000 public utilities. The EWG found a total of 260 contaminants, including 119 regulated chemicals, occurring in toxic amounts in our tap water. According to the EWG, the top 10 states with the highest contaminants in drinking water were (in order): California, Wisconsin, Arizona, Florida, North Carolina, Texas, New York, Nevada, Pennsylvania, and Illinois.

Even worse, in addition to the near impossibility of avoiding toxins in the water we cook with, drink, and bathe in, the very air we breathe is full of toxins, with indoor air being two to five times more polluted than outside air. This is true not only in states like Oregon, with an abundance of enormous, air-cleaning trees, but even in large cities. Our dwellings are no longer made of mud, straw, and other earth elements; they now are made of mostly chemically composed and/or treated products. The off-gassing of these is measurable, and detrimental to our health, and most of us do not have HEPA filters running in our homes and workplaces. And, let's not forget the commute. It's 90 degrees outside, and we shut ourselves into a metal can coated with toxins that have been heated. Think there isn't anything bad in that air? Or we open the windows, and breathe the exhaust fumes of the vehicles traveling with us. Yep, there's NASTY stuff in the air we breathe.

And that's not all. We also have to look at the toiletries we use, which are loaded with chemicals that are known neurotoxins and carcinogens. In the following chapters, you will get tips on how to reduce your toxic exposure, and how to detox your body.

On the same thread, in most cases (although the numbers are decreasing), babies are injected with toxic vaccines almost from the moment of birth, and then throughout their lives, if they follow mainstream practices. I have no intention of getting into a vaccine debate in this book, but an inarguable fact is that those vaccines contain numerous toxins. The cumulative effects of these are poorly studied, and will continue to be so as long as vaccination production is such a profitable industry.

The next prevalent toxin is DRUGS, DRUGS EVERYWHERE! According to the Mayo Clinic, 70 percent of Americans take prescription drugs, and more than half take at least two prescriptions regularly. Twenty percent of adults are on five or more prescription medications daily. Yes, prescription drugs can save lives, improve lives, and often be a very good choice. But the fact remains that they are not natural components to our bodies, and often contain compounds with harmful side effects. Most would agree that a preferable alternative would be to eliminate the situation requiring the drug rather than taking the drug. These medications often cause other symptoms that then require other drugs, and put us on a wheel of pharmaceuticals. These toxic compounds tax our body in uncountable ways while they are fixing a symptom. I would never tell a person to stop taking a drug. Instead, I recommend working to bring the body to a place where the drug is no longer needed, and then, in consultation with a medical provider, making an informed decision if, and when, a drug can be eliminated.

OH, BOY, the DIET is next. I honestly think it should have been first, but then you might have stopped reading. I mean, you can mess with the air I breathe, but not my pizza! It was hard for me to take food seriously, too. We all know we shouldn't eat junk food. But are we really WHAT WE EAT? Yes! Sad, frustrating, but true. You are what you eat. If you want to be a dead, round, black, flakey cookie filled with white, slimy, goo, then go for it. Eat the Oreo. Accept it, and adapt accordingly.

Through my self-study and self-care, I have had to eliminate a lot of foods that I like. Being raised by a single father, and having a mother who loved junk food, meant I grew up loving fast, easy, and cheap food with a big taste bang. I am now eating Vegan and grain free, with a few healthy exceptions (such as clean meat, or organic grain) once or twice a week. I recognize that it can very hard for some people to consider changing their diet. But, at some point, with sufficient motivation, it usually happens if you want to be well. On a day when my body was craving some chicken, I was standing at a deli counter. The server began telling me he could never go gluten free, or vegan, or give up the junk food he loves; he would rather die first. I calmly ignored his proclamations for several minutes, as he went on and on, until finally, he made eye contact with me, and I told him, "Well, I almost did!"

NO, I am NOT going to tell you what diet you should eat, nor am I qualified to do so. I really believe that every body is different, and each person's needs are different. But we are going to take some time and look into food, its effects on the body, and how you can go about designing the right diet for yourself. We are going to look at how to sort out which foods are making your body sick or simply weakening it. And we will look at what "power foods" might help you to be well.

Sometimes toxicity comes from the inside, and it's called "stinkin' thinkin'." The power of our mind and the thoughts that we generate is deeply underappreciated. When we create a negative thought in our mind, our body responds. When we create a positive thought in our mind, our body responds. If you don't believe me, take a few moments and create a REALLY happy scenario in your mind. Close your eyes, if it helps, and think of the sexiest moment you have ever experienced. Not into sexy experiences? Think of the saddest moment you have ever experienced. Did you notice changes in how your body feels? Now, try thinking of an experience that made you mad as HELL, and really think about it. Once again, notice how different your body feels. When we allow negative thoughts to become part of who we are, we are creating internal toxicity. We even begin to operate out of these lies about ourselves and our lives. Like the fight-or-flight response, our body doesn't distinguish between what is real, and what lives only in our thoughts – our body reacts as though our thoughts *are* real! Later in this book, I will give you practical ways to reverse this type of toxicity. I will equip you with ways to literally change your outlook by changing your inner thoughts.

I am going to call the next major stressor that can cause a decline in health LIFESTYLE, including sleep habits, exercise, and social life. First, let's look at sleep deprivation, or inadequate rest. For many modern people, our lifestyles are such that we rarely take time to rest. We wake up early and go to bed late, with much pressure in between to accomplish and succeed, all under a glorification of "busy-ness." The way we rush ourselves around and try to outdo each other with multi-tasking, you would think there was some reward for it. There is: we are wearing our bodies out! Our bodies need regular rest. Although sleep needs, like diets, are individual for each of us, the National Sleep Foundation's research has linked too-little sleep to a greater likelihood of obesity; increased risk of diabetes and heart disease; increased risk of depression, substance abuse, and other mental disorders; and practical problems like difficulty remembering things, concentrating, and paying attention. On the other side of the coin, there are many of us that have never built the habit of exercise (or at least do not do so now). This poor choice has dramatic effects on our sedentary culture. Since we no longer have to hand harvest our food, hike for water and build our own homes, we must create exercise in order to be well. "But I love to sleep!" you may say. Well, too much may be just as bad for you as too little. So, once again, the goal is moderation. Through the self-care outlined in this book, you may find that you will be sleeping better, and for a healthy duration.

Next, let's take on exercise. I bet you expect me to tell you to exercise more. Actually, I may suggest that you exercise less, believe it or not. In my line of work, I see many people who over-exercise. I have been guilty of over-exercising myself. Just as you know it is unhealthy for a person to work too much, it also is unhealthy to work out too much. Moderation in everything is key. Later in this book, we look at exercise, and how to gauge what amount and types are right for you.

How about a healthy social life? Well, if you are dealing with anxiety, social interactions may be really difficult for you. I know from experience. However, as you get healthier, you may find that you have less social anxiety and are more capable of having a healthy social life. On the other hand, maybe you have too much social life. I mean, are you the guy on Facebook posting half-naked pictures with drunken friends every weekend? We might want to address that, as well. Moderation, remember? If you're taking a couple of days to recover from your "social" weekend, that isn't encouraging good health, either.

Finally, you may think your declining health isn't your fault; it's in your GENES. Yes, we can't change what we were born with. We can't change our actual DNA, but we can change the habits that we inherited. Both of your parents may have diabetes, but that doesn't automatically mean you have to become diabetic. And if you do, that doesn't mean you have to suffer from it. I like to think of our genetics as being a predisposition toward something, rather than a sentence to it. Often, the reason a child ends up with a condition the parents had is because they grew up in the same house, eating the same food, learning the same habits, and believing the same reality would befall them because, after all, it's genetic. While I recognize that there is an unavoidable aspect of some inherited disease (as I mentioned, I have familial spinocerebellar ataxia, as does my mother), I also know that, all too often, living out those predispositions is a result of choices. For instance, if I had grown up eating the type of diet I feed my children, it's likely I would have avoided some of my health challenges. With the Internet, and the instant availability of information in today's world, we have far greater power than our parents did when it comes to learning how to be healthy, and taking care of ourselves and our children.

What I hope to do in this book is to show you that good health is not dependent on just one thing. The body, mind, and spirit all work together, and each and every bodily system relies on the others to support it. We are very intricate beings, wonderfully and beautifully made. Caring for ourselves is of utmost importance when it comes to living at our full potential. Only with a strong body, mind, and spirit can we rise up and be all that we are capable of.

Although what we've examined so far could be seen as "doom and gloom," with little or no hope to de-stress and de-toxify our lives and our environment, I hope you will see more. See that although we live in a toxic world, there is hope. We are going to move through together, step by step, and look at how you can take charge of your wellbeing, and gain or regain vitality.

Down in the Ditch

I remember one of my "lower than low" times. Actually, it seemed for a few years like those were all I had. During that time, I felt like my whole life was going in a different direction than I had ever dreamed or planned. It was as if the new direction had no hope, no light, and no power in it. Depression consumed me, and it seemed I couldn't muster a thought that wasn't "stinkin' thinkin'." And then a song came on the radio that really spoke to me. Wynonna Judd sang me a truth that I needed to hear in a song called *'Rock Bottom'*. (No wise cracks about liking country music. I was raised in Texas!)

Whether you are a country music aficionado or not, it would be hard to argue with the truth in the song. The great thing about being in the ditch is that it's a perfect place to count the stars. Once I had my fun with the pity party and let go of my attachments to my plans for my life, I found a good deal of peace and was able to make a choice to turn things around. I was going to feel better, be healthier, and live happier, and it was all up to ME.

To be completely honest, though, I stayed in that ditch long enough to begin to get comfortable there. I mean, I knew I was going to get up eventually, but there was warmth and shelter in the ditch. I began to like the familiarity of being sick and pathetic. Of course, I wouldn't admit that at the time, but I was able to see it eventually. I realized anything that becomes familiar breeds a certain amount of comfort. In other words, there's comfort in the familiar, even when the familiar is uncomfortable.

One of the good things about staying in the ditch is there isn't much risk. There isn't much fear of loss, and you can see things coming right at you. Plus, let's face it, you can't get any lower. Besides that, no one really expects too much of you if they know you are in the ditch. You really don't expect much of yourself, either, so there is less pressure. I fully recognize that taking shelter in the ditch helped me, in some ways, to heal my spirit. I had a lot of quiet time in the ditch, and that seemed to soothe my soul. But the ditch is no place to make a home, is it?!

One of the problems with the ditch is that it is hard to climb out of. Certainly, it is harder to climb out of a ditch than it is to get up off of flat ground. It takes effort, and there is even the risk of falling back in. Let's face it; it is easier just to stay there, isn't it?

Another problem is that when we're in the ditch, we often can get sympathy and nurturing we really need from people. The need for sympathy and nurturing may be a void in our lives that we're seeking to fill. If those needs are being met when we're in the ditch, that can make it hard to want to leave. The healthy solution would be to sort out better ways to get that kind of attention without having to be sick to get it. The first place to start is with honesty. My first marriage was with a man who was great in many ways, but had NO ability to nurture. We often joked that if I ever became seriously ill, I was screwed (not too funny now, I guess). I am now married to an incredibly nurturing man (more nurturing than I am, actually), and in the beginning of our relationship, he filled a huge void. His love and nurturing covered years of need, and still continue to do so. However, there was a point when I recognized there was the tiniest bit of me that would regret feeling better because I would lose some of his nurturing.

I had to be real with myself, and face what I would lose and what I would gain by healing myself. I recommend you do the same. By facing my unspoken (and sometimes imagined) fears, I was able to extinguish them by offering more positive solutions. I found other things that could replace the type of nurturing a sick person receives, like having energy to go out on dates with my husband, and enjoying being lively with him.

French poet and novelist Anatole France said it well:
All changes, even the most longed for, have their melancholy; for what we leave behind us is a part of ourselves; we must die to one life before we can enter another.

By taking a good, hard look at where we are, and why we are there, we can begin to formulate a plan to move forward and begin healing our body, mind, and spirit.

Action Steps:

- Write a whole page about where you are in life in relation to the ditch and why you are there.
- Make a list of the pros and cons of being right where you are, right now. What are you getting by staying in the ditch (both positive and negative)? What are you missing?
- Then make a list of the pros and cons of healing yourself. What will you gain? What will you lose?

It's in Your Quality of Mind

We are going to delve into aspects of the mind now, and I am going to share with you some teachings from yoga. The ancient teachings of yoga are vast, and begin with the training of an individual's character. From there, one moves into the qualities of the mind and our motivations. Yoga refers to three qualities of the mind, called **gunas**. First, there is **tamas,** which is translated as inertia, dullness, lethargy. Second, there is **sattva,** which is translated as creativity, clarity, or harmony - which is our aim, and considered the steady point. Third, there is **rajas,** which is translated as activity or movement, and is necessary when making a change.

While each quality is, in and of itself, a healthy place to visit, it is sattva where we want to make our "home" - our main state of being. When we have the need to make change, rajas is essential. Without it, we would surely stay in the ditch. When we over-exert ourselves, or burn ourselves out, tamas will allow us the rest necessary to heal. So, both rajas and tamas have their place, and both ultimately are a part of bringing us to a state of sattva.

Tamas is the way nature destroys or completes things. Although we need tamas to help us rest and sleep, excessive tamas dulls the mind, making us lazy, inert, and depressed. People with an excessively tamasic nature often engage in a self-destructive lifestyle and diet. They tend to be gluttonous, eating, drinking, and having sex excessively. It's common for these individuals to consume alcohol and other drugs in large quantities. As the tamasic mind becomes dull, heavy, and confused, the individual becomes increasingly less caring about herself/himself and others. The mind may become so dull that the individual is unable to articulate clearly, and needs assistance in making decisions.

When a person's mind is absorbed in tamas, they will truly need help, as their ability to discriminate between what is beneficial, and what is not, is weak. The mind has become so unclear, it cannot be trusted to make healthy decisions.

Individuals who are dealing with illness and disease most often are dealing with excessive tamas (although some lean toward rajas, as discussed below). Therefore, a balance must be created. Creating this balance will take work, and it will be uncomfortable, but it is all in your power.

If you lean toward too much tamas, it will take rajas to pull yourself out of the ditch and dust yourself off. Rajas is essential to move you away from tamas, and ultimately to rest in sattva. It will take rajas to get you to put your boots on and pull yourself up - to make changes that will heal your body, your mind, and your spirit, and make yourself well

On the other hand, imbalanced ***rajas*** leads to excessive pride, competitiveness, aggression, and jealousy. People with a lot of rajas tend to value power, prestige, and material success.

People with rajasic temperaments may tend towards fanaticism. They hold their beliefs very strongly, trying to convert others, sometimes at the expense of relationships. There is often chaotic activity and drama surrounding them, and their minds are so full they don't really listen to any advice, even if they request it. Excessive exercise to the point of over-exertion is rajasic, and disturbing to the body, mind, and spirit systems. Excessive thinking, working, talking, travelling, or any kind of over-stimulation, also is overly rajasic.

However, rajas is essential to achieving any kind of goal, and is healthy in moderation. If you lean toward too much rajas, then it is going to be tamas that will help bring you into balance, or sattva. You will have to learn to slow down, quiet down. and simply do less.

Sattva is clear, creative, and manifests life. Peace, harmony, love, and truth are all sattvic qualities. People who are predominantly sattvic tend to be quietly spiritual and steady in their faith, without being fanatical. These people are humble, content, happy, and not easily angered. Their minds are sharp, and their perceptions are clear. They are pleasant, inspiring, curious, and creative. Sattva represents the steady middle ground between tamas and rajas.

Here are some actions you can take and foods you can eat to cultivate the needed quality of mind to heal you.

Tamasic foods are lacking in life force, and do not support energy. These include old and leftover food; deeply fried food; and excessive meat, chicken, seafood, eggs, and hard cheeses. Alcohol and other drugs may be either tamasic or rajasic, depending on the type and amount consumed.

To balance tamas means clearing out the cobwebs in the brain. Fresh air, peaceful yet dynamic exercise, and sattvic foods, lifestyle, and environment will help balance tamas.

Rajasic foods stimulate and irritate the system. Junk foods like potato chips and chocolate, and salty, excessively sweet, pungent, or spicy foods (like raw onions and garlic), can agitated and disturb the mind. Most legumes and beans increase rajas slightly, and they should be soaked prior to consuming.

To balance rajas means limiting our exposure to foods, people, and situations that disturb our minds, and increasing our exposure to more sattvic foods, lifestyle, and people. Anything that increases sattva will decrease rajas. Recognize that if you are rajas dominant, you can utilize some of the healthy aspects of tamas to bring you toward healing. Likewise, if you are tamas-dominant, utilize healthy aspects of rajas to bring you to healing.

Sattvic foods are full of life force, easy to digest, and light, such as lightly-cooked organic vegetables; ripe fruit, nuts, and seeds; raw honey; ginger; fennel seeds; cardamom; and small amounts of ghee (clarified butter). Pure cow's milk is considered sattvic, if taken from cows raised humanely. If dairy doesn't agree with you, alternative nut or grain milk is acceptable.

To increase sattva, we also need to engage in sattvic activities. These could include listening to relaxing and uplifting music, walking in a peaceful environment, and practicing Gentle Yoga (my favorite), pranayama, meditation, tai chi, or chi gong. Another very simple way to entice a sattvic quality is to limit your exposure to stressful and/or negative people and situations.

WHEW. That was a lot of new information for most of us! You can think of it this way: we know in our culture that many people tend to be either "hyper," driven workaholics, or unemployed, depressed, and hopeless. In the middle are those lucky people who are happy, healthy, and well-balanced. The teachings of yoga have recognized this for thousands of years, and break it down in a very clear way into the three *gunas*. For optimal health, we all need to strive for a balance of tamas, rajas, and sattva, knowing all the while that we will oscillate back and forth from one end of the spectrum to the other.

There was a time in my life when I called myself a perfectionist. Everything had to be "just so," or I would not be happy. Those were my 20s. It was a time of having babies, and proving that I was the best darned homemaker and mother in the whole world. Then there were my 30s, when I spent four years as a single mom, home-schooling four children, and about lost my flipping mind. I learned to cultivate qualities of tamas, and unfortunately, I didn't stop. I went overboard with tamas, and my health declined dramatically. Since then, it has been a process of bringing myself to sattva and creating an environment of healing.

The power of the mind cannot be understated when it comes to the condition of our health. In order to heal ourselves, we must address the qualities of the mind, and cultivate a quality conducive to healing.

Action Steps:

- Determine your dominant quality of mind.
- List activities and/or foods you can add to your life to bring you toward *sattva*.
- List activities and/or foods you can eliminate from your life to bring you toward *sattva*.

A Decision Has to be Made

There is an aspect of this whole concept of healing yourself that we have to look at seriously. The question I would ask you is, "Do you WANT to be well, or do you just WISH you were well?"

Antoine de Saint-Exupéry said, *"A goal without a plan is just a wish."*

Now is the point when you have to be honest with yourself about whether you are only wishing to be well, or you are making a decision to heal yourself. Somewhere, deep within yourself, you must come a decision - a decision to make a change and to take charge of your future. In order to begin healing, you must decide you are no longer going to accept the path you are on, and realize that you are the only one who can truly change the course of your life.

When I first started to be clearly ill, I went to multiple doctors and had many tests. It was at a time when I was experiencing secondary infertility and miscarriages, and I was depressed. I was 25 years old, and I can remember, in vivid detail, the smell of the office, the look of the room, and the feel of the chair I sat on when the doctor told me I was in the early stages of lupus. He proceeded to tell me what to expect in my future. At that point, I drew inward. It was like a fog, like someone was playing a movie in front of me that I wasn't watching. By the time he finished speaking, an internal fire was ablaze. I was infuriated that I was there. I was infuriated that he was telling me this. I was infuriated that I let myself get to this point of losing faith and trust in my body. I was infuriated that I had lost the deep belief that our minds and spirits create the body we live in. I said nothing, other than to thank him calmly, and I left and never went back. Something inside of me had changed.

Because of this fury that I felt, I was propelled into learning how to heal myself. I did not accept that it was impossible for me to heal myself. Somewhere in my young life, a belief had been instilled in me that our bodies are miraculous, and if we give them the right elements and put them in the right environment, they will heal. I did regain my health, and enjoyed good health for several years.

However, as the stress of my life and the choices I made began to wear on me, I once again became sick. I was beaten down; I was broken and ill. Along that path, I lost the belief that my body was miraculous. I gave up trying to heal myself, and I looked outside of my own power for healing. During this time, I spent years trying different body work and healing modalities, in the hope that they would be the magic, missing element, and one of them could make me well. Each and every thing I tried was good, but wasn't IT. No one could make me well. When I realized I was going to have to take charge and find the spark within myself once again, I wasn't sure I could muster it. I found myself with the realization that my future had two possibilities - one of disease and hopelessness, and one of empowerment and vitality – and I knew I HAD to make a choice to get up and heal myself.

For a while, I pitied myself for the fact that I have to work so darned hard at being well. But once I just accepted that I may have not been gifted with wellness, but I sure could earn it, I settled in. Thankfully, I already knew becoming well wouldn't be a fast-track, and the journey would be life-long.

I'll share with you a closing quote for this chapter:

Singer-songwriter Tori Amos says, "Healing takes courage, and we all have courage, even if we have to dig a little to find it." I encourage you to dig a little, and find the courage to step onto the path toward healing.

Action Step:

- Make a decision to heal yourself, and write it down. Post it on your refrigerator.

The Path of Healing

Gaining this understanding has brought me enormous peace. Even though I tend to be an impatient person, I've learned to appreciate that it is the actual journey that makes us ready to be at our destination. In a literal way, this gave me the ability to understand that even though I had a goal of being healthy and active, it would take a while. I also was able to understand that the journey might not be easy. Another aspect of keeping my eyes on the path before me was coming to understood that I could not expect myself to be capable of being healthy and active until I had sorted out every aspect of creating a healthy body, mind, and spirit – a process that would take a lot of learning and practice.

In addition, this understanding gave me the freedom to enjoy the path, and enjoy the resting spots along the way, all the while knowing that resting or taking breaks in no way meant I was quitting.

For example, looking back, I recall when I first gave up gluten. My health improved dramatically and I was excited, confident that I would reach my goal soon! However, I wasn't there yet. I was left with leaky gut, and many imbalances because of it, and needed to take the time and energy to heal these things. At first, my natural tendency was to be impatient or discouraged, but I remembered that the path to health and vitality is a long one, and I was able to recognize what I had fixed already.

Through my days in network marketing, I learned another great analogy for goals and paths. This analogy uses an airplane. We all know a plane sets out with a specific destination, but what you may not know is that the plane is only on course about 10% of the time. The remaining 90% of the time, it is correcting its course. Yet, the plane usually reaches its destination, at or near the expected time. Knowing this can be an encouragement for us in life, as well. We don't have to be spot-on all the time. Sometimes, taking one step reveals to us that it was not a step we needed to take, but we would never know that until we took the step.

What it takes to continue on your path is commitment and persistence. You can't just set up permanent camp when you have not reached our destination. If you are a person who lacks persistence, I recommend you find a way to encourage yourself. For some people, rewards are a great incentive. When it comes to your path, only you will know what rewards would be good for you. And only you will know what milestones to set as achievement points.

An important way to fuel your persistence is by feeding your body, mind, and spirit - all three. You will need to find things and take actions that will nourish every aspect of your being in order to have the strength to continue down your path. We will discuss specific actions later in this book.

Action Steps:

- Create in your mind's eye an image of what a "healthy you" would look and feel like.
- Write down a description of this image/goal.

Study

This is not a topic that everyone gets excited about. In addition, our society conditions us to let the 'medical professionals' do our thinking for us. We have been taught to simply trust their learning and experience, and let them decide what is going on with our bodies and what our bodies need. I will tell you right now, that is going to have to change if you are going to heal yourself.

Most of us - likely including you, because you are reading this book - have given the doctors more than a fair chance to heal us. We probably have exhausted every avenue of medical wisdom, to little or no avail. To be honest, I have vacillated back and forth multiple times in my 20 years of working to heal myself, going from that place where I am looking at others to 'fix' me, and the place where I know I am the one who has to heal myself. I'm sure you aren't surprised when I say it is the latter that actually has healed me. It has been me, utilizing my own power, that has made me well.

The LARGEST tool in my doing so has been study – the kind of hard-core, concentrated reading and research that can make your mind go numb. My studies typically would begin with searching about symptoms I was experiencing, and continuing to search and study about causes and possible solutions, all the while attempting to discern what seemed to be true for me and my body. When I had diagnoses, obviously it then would involve studying about those specific conditions. The biggest chunk of my study has been about how to make the body the most clean and strong as it possibly can be. I've studied about diet, fitness, rest, holistic and naturopathic treatments, and everything else I could think of that might play a part in my health.

One purpose of this book is to take some of the work out of the study aspect for you. The approach I will be presenting to you is a holistic and rounded way to support every bodily system and heal you. However, you shouldn't consider it the "end all" to being well. I encourage you to do a good deal of studying and research about your own conditions, and apply what you learn in order to have the greatest advantage to healing yourself.

Another aspect of study that I know will be invaluable to you is called svadhyaya in Sanskrit, and it means "self-study." Svadhyaya encompasses the whole idea of getting to know YOU, what motivates your thoughts, feelings, and insecurities, and working to peel back the layers until you get to the real, authentic you. This YOU that you are looking for is the one who hasn't been hurt or disappointed. It's the one who can feel and express love freely, toward yourself and others. This is the YOU who doesn't suffer from stress or pain, because you have shed the useless layers that you create in your mind. I encourage you to do self-study, and in order to do so, you may want to have a teacher or study group that has a plan for self-study. Another good way to do this is through reading of good books on character development, and through journaling.

This study will take time, and until you have that time in your life, you likely won't get far on your path to heal yourself. You will need to look honestly at your life, and consider whether you have time to read about the things you will be involved in to heal yourself. If you cannot prioritize sufficient time for self-study, then it is unrealistic to expect that you will be able to heal yourself. Nevertheless, that doesn't mean you shouldn't start down the path; it will just take you longer. This may be a wakeup call that you need to adjust your life to make time to devote to healing yourself.

With the help of this book, you will be able to create a path for yourself that will lead to healing and increased vitality. Remember that not everyone can expect to achieve 100% healing, but by taking these steps and walking down your path, you will generate better health and increased vitality. In the end, you will have a pretty clear picture of what your goal looks like, and what the path ahead of you looks like, but know that your journey can change slightly and adapt as you go.

Action Steps:

- Evaluate your schedule and the amount of time you can devote to study.
- Expect to need a minimum of three to six hours a week to do this.

Heal Your Body

In order to heal yourself, you must heal all three natures of YOU. These would be the body, mind, and spirit. To heal only one of these could create minimal healing, but to heal all three is to create lasting and deep healing. The synergy created by harmonizing the body, mind, and spirit can't be overstated.

Reduce Stress

Near the beginning of this book, we talked about the causes of decline in our health. We will revisit those again here, beginning with stress. Stress is linked to the six leading causes of death. The good news is that, for the most part, stress is actually something we can control. In fact, aside from actual structural stressors (for example, stress on soft tissue caused by a broken bone or other injury, or illness), I propose that every stress we experience is our own creation! Of course, every unique situation that causes stress is capable of producing different results, and some situations obviously are harder to control than others. Nevertheless, whatever degree of stress we experience, it is our *thoughts* that create the stress. For example, imagine that my hair began falling out, and I was feeling very stressed about this. Where would the stress come from? It would come from my thoughts about the situation. I might think I will look ugly, and be concerned about how others will react to my appearance. I may worry that losing my hair means I am very sick and won't attain good health. All of these thoughts are what causes the stress. Because stress comes from our thoughts about a situation, we can change our thoughts and reduce our stress. We are in control! That is good news.

With my choice to continue home-schooling following my divorce, I realized that I had to change the way I thought about it. I had to frame the situation in my mind in a way that would create less stress. I had to get even more organized and quite a bit more relaxed. It took about a year before I realized that I had never even heard of anyone else attempting to be a single parent and home-school on their own. Knowing this helped me to lighten up and give myself a break.

Prior to my divorce, I was a fastidious homemaker. I liked things in order and clean, and I could not relax unless they were. As I found myself adjusting to being a single mom, I found it quite impossible to keep things the way I wanted them in my home. The way I saw it was that I could either completely exhaust myself keeping things to my previous standards of living, or I could change my standards of living. I chose the second, and learned that, lo and behold, dust and dirty floors cannot kill me! Now, do I look forward to one day having a perfectly clean home all the time? YES. But I know when that time comes, I also will miss my children.

As a yoga practitioner and teacher, my most valued lesson is just this very topic.
Well-known author and motivational speaker Wayne Dyer, Ph.D. says, "If you change the way you look at things, the things you look at change." Maybe even more to the point I am making here, graphic artist Mary Engelbreit says it a different way: "If you don't like something, change it; if you can't change it, change the way you think about it."

To understand the effects of stress on the body, we will look at the nervous system. The nervous system consists of the central nervous system (CNS) (the brain and spinal cord), and the peripheral nervous system (PNS), which connects the CNS to the other parts of the body. The PNS includes the somatic nervous system, which controls voluntary movement, and the autonomic nervous system (ANS), which largely controls involuntary functions like digestion, breathing, and heart rate. Within the ANS, there are three main sub-systems: the sympathetic nervous system (SNS) (the "fight or flight" system), the parasympathetic nervous system (PNS) (the "rest and recover" system), and the enteric nervous system (which controls the gastrointestinal tract). Our focus here is on the SNS and the PNS. Both of those systems are necessary to our health and safety, but one is conducive to our health and helping us to heal, while the other is responsible for keeping us safe in a crisis.

The SNS is responsible for saving us when danger is looming. It causes internal changes to the automatic nervous system, such as increasing heart rate, producing adrenaline, slowing digestion, and sharpening vision. All of these changes come together to prepare a body to fight or flee, and they are in no way conducive to healing. In fact, if the body stays in this heightened state long enough, it will break down.

The PNS is the one responsible for calming us and healing us. It slows the heart rate and blood pressure, increases digestion, and allows us to feel at peace. This is the state in which our body should be naturally, and is the state in which healing can occur.

We know stress is detrimental to our health, and that when the SNS is in control, our bodies are compromised physically. Therefore, in order to heal, we MUST learn to manage stress, and promote a state that induces the PNS. What is both great and awful about the nervous system is that it loves habit. Therefore, if you frequently go to one system or the other, the body will begin switching to that familiar system more easily. If you routinely stimulate your SNS with your habits and patterns of thinking, then your body happily will put you there at the slightest encouragement. Happily, the same is true for the PNS. We must learn to make a habit out of stimulating the healthier nervous system. In a moment, I will give you a simple exercise to do just that. But first, let's look at some of the warning signs and symptoms of stress:

Cognitive Symptoms
- Memory problems
- Inability to concentrate
- Poor judgment
- Seeing only the negative
- Anxious or racing thoughts
- Constant worrying

Emotional Symptoms
- Moodiness
- Irritability or short temper
- Agitation
- Inability to relax
- Feeling overwhelmed
- Sense of loneliness and isolation
- Depression or general unhappiness

Physical Symptoms
- Aches and pains
- Diarrhea or constipation
- Nausea, dizziness
- Chest pain, rapid heartbeat
- Loss of sex drive
- Frequent colds

Behavioral Symptoms

- Eating more or less
- Sleeping too much or too little
- Isolating yourself from others
- Procrastinating or neglecting responsibilities
- Using alcohol, cigarettes, or other drugs to relax
- Nervous habits (e.g., nail biting, pacing)

If you have three or more of these symptoms, you probably have a detrimental level of stress in your life that needs to be eliminated. So, how can you do that? The obvious would be to sort out what is causing the stress, and either change it or get rid of it. If that is not possible, then change the way you view that situation.

Action Step:

- Identify situations that cause you stress, and choose to either change the situations or change the way you think about them.
- When people get on your nerves, assume the best of them, and don't let them steal your peace.
- Daily, take 10 minutes to be quiet, and breathe deeply. Doing this THREE times a day is optimal. Once a day is a good start.
- You can immediately induce the PNS with a simple exercise. This exercise works every time without fail. Use a yoga block, a thickly-folded blanket, a pillow, or any object you can place beneath your pelvis to elevate your hips 3-5 inches off of a surface you will lie on (if you are obese, stay around 3 inches in elevation). At this height, the exercise is safe for everyone. Some find that the most comfortable option is to place a block on the floor, and lay a folded blanket over the block in a way that it will create a ramp for your back low back. Lie on

your back, with this prop under your pelvis, and bending your knees with the soles of your feet on the floor. Place a small, rolled towel under your neck. Rest your arms at your sides, palms up, with enough space between your arms and your body to create space in your arm pits. Take deep, slow breaths. Rest here with your eyes closed for a minimum of 5-10 minutes, twice a day. This will active your PNS immediately, encouraging you to feel more peaceful, and generating your natural energy. Make sure you don't skimp on the time, as it takes four minutes for the PNS to kick in. When you prepare to rise, roll onto your right side, taking a couple of breaths before you gently push yourself up. If you have varicose veins, or simply want even more benefit from a greater inversion, elevate your feet during this exercise by propping them on a bed, couch, or wall. However, if you have uncontrolled high blood pressure or glaucoma, or are menstruating, don't elevate your feet.

Rid Yourself of Toxins

In his 2010 article "Is There Toxic Waste In Your Body," Mark Hyman, M.D. presents some alarming statistics about our exposure to environmental toxins. According to Dr. Hyman, each of us is exposed to 6 million pounds of mercury, and 2.5 billion pounds of other toxic chemicals, each year! He goes on to state:

> *Eighty thousand toxic chemicals have been released into our environment since the dawn of the industrial revolution, and very few have been tested for their long-*

term impact on human health. And let me tell you, the results aren't pretty for those that have been tested. . . .

How can we not be affected by this massive amount of poison?

According to the nonprofit organization Environmental Working Group, the average newborn baby has 287 known toxins in his or her umbilical cord blood.

If a newborn is exposed to that many toxins, imagine how many you have been exposed to in your life. . . .

In order to heal the body, we must stop the toxic assault on the body. Let's go through the most accessible ways to do this.

Many of the foods we eat are loaded with cancer-causing poisons, applied in the name of pest control. Unless we eat strictly organic, we are taking in chemicals that cause cancer, dementia, and more. Minimally, they assault the immune system and clog the liver. Often, they attack the nervous system. If you want to heal yourself, it is essential that switch to organic foods wherever possible, and seize every opportunity to choose meats from animals that are free-range, grass-fed, and humanely raised. I KNOW it's more expensive! But the more we consumers demand organic foods by purchasing them, the more the cost will go down. Your health is infinitely too valuable to buy cheap food. **Go organic.**

Water is the next big source of toxic exposure. Switch to a good filter, and I don't mean the ones you buy at Walmart. And, no, bottled water is not an option. There have been enough reports to show the toxicity of bottled water that it should only be used in emergency situations. Do not drink bottled water! You will need to filter not only your drinking water, but the water you bathe in, as well. Unfortunately, price is a good gauge of quality in this realm, so don't skimp. Personally, my family uses the water systems from Nikken. Pay now and reap the benefit of better health. ***Filter your water.***

The indoor air we breathe is said to be two to five times more polluted than outside air. Because we eliminate more waste through our lungs than we do by sweating, urinating, and defecating combined, we should put much more emphasis than we currently do on the quality of the air we breathe. Again, the same thing applies to air filters as to water filters: you get what you pay for. Again, my family uses an air filter from Nikken, and we have seen amazing things with it, such as my daughter's eczema going away and improvement in food sensitivities. If you can only afford one system, then put it in your bedroom; you spend more time there than anywhere else. If possible, get one for where you work, as well. ***Filter your air.***

We also have to look at the toiletries we use, most of which are loaded with chemicals that are recognized neurotoxins and carcinogens.

CANCERactive, a Britain cancer charity, lists dozens of toxic chemicals found in everyday products. In their article "12 Common Toiletries and their chemicals of concern" the group reported that toothpaste, deodorants, shampoo and conditioner, shaving products, lipstick, shower gels and liquid soaps, foundation, hairspray, hair dyes, mouthwash, nail polish, and talcum powder/baby powder, all contain chemicals which, in high doses, are deemed carcinogenic and neurotoxic, and cause mutation of DNA. While the doses of these chemicals may be minimal in a particular product, the European community has already banned 1,000 or more of these chemicals, ordering that they be replaced with safer alternatives – a process that could take up to fifteen years to complete.

So, you can see there are many things we do to ourselves to create toxic exposure. You undoubtedly can find many more items in your home, such as cleaning supplies, that should be replaced with natural products. This is an area where your study and research will be helpful. You can find almost limitless information on Pinterest for making your own natural products – a fun and cost effective solution. ***Replace toxic toiletries and household products.***

Action Steps:

- Go organic
- Filter water
- Filter air
- Replace toiletries and household products with all natural ones

The 5 Organs of Elimination

By this point, you have stopped the toxic assault on your body, and are ready to start cleaning house - and by "house," I mean the body you live in. Most of us either own, or have owned, a car, and know the filters need to be replaced in order for the vehicle to run smoothly. The same is true for our body. The colon, liver, kidneys, lungs, and skin are the five organs of elimination, and they are vitally important to keep clean. It is essential that you first stop the onslaught of toxicity, and then cleanse your organs of elimination, before you ever do any detoxification.

Detox programs and diets are all the rage right now, and that, in and of itself, is good. What is bad is that people take their toxic bodies and their toxic five organs of elimination, and do a detox that floods these systems with even more waste. Due to the congested or weakened state of any or all of these systems, the body often can't handle a detox very well, and can become quite sick from a detox.

While I am a firm believer in doing regular diet detoxes, and we will discus this in future sections, I insist that we must cleanse and support the organs of elimination prior to and during a detox.

I recommend starting with cleansing *the colon first*. There are many great colon cleanses on the market, and I suggest going to your local health food store and getting guidance. Cleanses from ReNew Life have worked well for me. The company has a complete line of cleanses, from a basic cleanse to parasite cleanses and yeast cleanses. However, everyone's body responds differently, so be present to your own body's reactions to cleanses you try, and find what works best for you.

It's said that at any given point in time, at least 80% of the population has a parasite. If you are sick, it is likely that you have a parasite and/or yeast overgrowth. Therefore, it's worth your time to read about these other cleanses, and decide if doing these additional colon cleanses makes sense for you.

Here are some symptoms of intestinal parasites:

- You have unexplained constipation, diarrhea, gas, or other symptoms of IBS
- You traveled internationally, and remember getting traveler's diarrhea while abroad

- You have a history of food poisoning, and your digestion has not been the same since.
- You have trouble falling asleep, or you wake up multiple times during the night.
- You get skin irritations or unexplained rashes, hives, rosacea, or eczema.
- You grind your teeth in your sleep.
- You have pain or aching in your muscles or joints.
- You experience fatigue, exhaustion, depression, or frequent feelings of apathy.
- You never feel satisfied or full after your meals.
- You've been diagnosed with iron-deficiency anemia.

Candida albicans is a common yeast that exists in everyone's body. However, when this yeast becomes overgrown, it can manifest in many symptoms and cause a host of diseases, as well as worsen whatever other health challenges you have.

You may ask how you get candida overgrowth. The healthy bacteria in your gut generally keep your candida levels at an acceptable level. However, there are several factors that can cause the candida population to get out of hand:

- Eating a diet high in refined carbohydrates and sugars
- Excessive consumption of otherwise-beneficial fermented foods, like kombucha, kefir, sauerkraut. and pickles
- Excessive consumption of alcohol
- Oral contraceptives
- High-stress lifestyle
- Antibiotics and corticosteroids

Certain illnesses and conditions also can make candida infection more likely, including uncontrolled diabetes, HIV infection, cancer, dry mouth/dehydration, and hormonal changes that occur during pregnancy.

The following are possible symptoms of candidiasis (candida overgrowth):

- Oral Thrush
- Low sex drive
- Recurring vaginal yeast infections
- Migraine headaches
- Sinus, ear, or eye infections
- Toenail fungus
- Skin fungus
- Adrenal fatigue
- Rashes, including jock itch
- Food allergies
- Brain fog
- Depression
- Just plain feeling "whacked out" and irritated
- Fatigue
- Low thyroid

My favorite self-test for candida overgrowth is the spit test. Basically, you spit in a glass of water first thing in the morning, before eating, drinking, or brushing teeth. There are several outcomes for the appearance of the saliva. For instance, the saliva, itself, may float, while "strings" of yeast colonies may extend down into the water after a few minutes. Or the saliva may be very cloudy, and begin sinking to the bottom of the glass. You can Google "candida spit test" to get further information and images.

The majority of people who are sick or are eating a typical American diet will have candidiasis, and you should consider doing a candida cleanse. I love the book "The Candida Cure:

Yeast, Fungus & Your Health, The 90-Day Program to Beat Candida & Restore Vibrant Health," by Ann Boroch (rev. 2014).

For me, candida not only was contributing to my gut health, but it also likely was affecting my joints. Candida can invade absolutely any body tissue, and although it isn't easy to get rid of, the result is a huge impact on healing your body. *Cleanse your colon.*

Cleansing **the liver** should be next, and will give you a big bang for your buck, so to speak. The liver's primary job is to filter and detoxify the blood that comes from the digestive tract, before moving it to the rest of the body. The liver breaks down chemicals and metabolizes drugs so they can be excreted. While it does this, the liver secretes bile that ends up back in the intestines. In addition, the liver makes proteins essential to blood clotting and other functions. Cleansing the liver allows it to perform all of these functions more efficiently. Again, I personally have used liver cleanse products from ReNew Life, but there are many quality products on the market. Adding red clover and/or dandelion root teas will assist a liver cleanse, as will taking artichoke, either in capsules or by consuming plant itself. When it comes to the liver, everyone needs to do this cleanse, especially before doing a whole body detox. *Cleanse your liver.*

The kidneys also need cleansing and support regularly, and especially prior to a total body detox. The kidneys' function is to filter the blood. All of our blood passes through the kidneys several times a day. The kidneys control the body's fluid balance, regulate the balance of electrolytes, and remove wastes. As the kidneys filter blood, they create urine, which drains down tubes called ureters to the bladder. Several effective kidney cleanses are available on the market. *Cleanse your kidneys.*

When it comes to cleansing **the lungs**, it is pretty simple: breathe deeply, and take or eat rosemary, which has been found to increase circulation to the capillaries in the lungs. When you breathe deeply, you are exercising and cleaning your lungs. Do 10 minutes of deep breathing daily, in a clean environment. However, avoid breathing at more than 90% of your lung capacity, as you can create scar tissue in the lungs by over-extending them repeatedly. Your deep breathing could be done while you are resting with your hips elevated to stimulate the PNS, as discussed above in the "Reduce Stress" section. You may recall that we eliminate more waste through our breathing than through urinating, sweating, and defecating combined, so take this step seriously. *Cleanse your lungs.*

Your skin is your largest organ, and protects you from the world that you live in. Skin performs many different roles, including production of vitamin D, protection, excretion, temperature regulation, and sensation.

Your skin has many receptors (sensors) that perceive sensations such as touch, temperature changes, pressure, and pain. Skin protects you against exposure to dangerous things in the environment such as bacteria. It also repels water, minimizes water loss from the body, and protects underlying structures such as blood vessels, nerves, and organs.

Your skin helps you maintain a healthy body temperature by changing the diameter of the blood vessels in the dermis. In addition, to cool your body, blood vessels in the skin enlarge in diameter so that heat is lost through the skin. When warmth is needed, the blood vessel diameters become smaller, and heat is conserved
through sweating.

Your body excretes substances through the skin. First is sebum (skin oil), which helps in making your skin water repellent and smooth in texture, and also defends your body against fungus and bacteria. In addition, water, salts, and several other substances are excreted from the skin, through the process of perspiration. When you are exposed to ultraviolet light from the sun, your body produces Vitamin D, which is an essential vitamin needed to keep the body healthy. Thus, the skin is a vital organ of elimination.

The first way to cleanse the skin is to eat and drink clean food and water. Another great cleansing technique is to do dry brushing. These are some of the benefits of dry brushing:

- Helps with muscle tone and gives you a more even distribution of fat deposits.
- Increases the circulation to the skin, which can reduce the appearance of cellulite, a toxic material accumulated in your body's fat cells.
- Rejuvenates the nervous system by stimulating nerve endings in the skin.
- Helps remove dead skin cells (and encourage cell renewal), which results in smoother and brighter skin.
- Assists in improving vascular blood circulation and lymphatic drainage. By releasing toxins, it encourages the body's discharge of metabolic wastes so the body is able to run more effectively.
- Helps your skin to absorb nutrients by eliminating clogged pores.

Here's how you do it:

- Obtain a high-quality, natural-bristle brush. Bristles should be of medium stiffness. A long handle is helpful for reaching your entire back.
- Perform dry brushing on dry skin, immediately before showering.
- Work in gentle, circular, upward motions, and then longer, smoother strokes. Pressure should be firm, but not painful.
- Always begin at the ankles and work upward towards the heart. The lymphatic fluid flows through the body towards the heart, so it's important that you brush in the same direction.
- Your back is the only exception to the preceding rule; brush from the neck down to the lower back.
- After you've finished with the ankles, move up to the lower legs, thighs, stomach, back, and arms. Be cautious over softer and sensitive skin around the chest and breasts, and never brush your genitals, or any areas with varicose veins, inflammation, sores or abrasions, sunburn, or skin cancer.
- Brushing your face is acceptable, but requires a soft bristled brush.
- Shower promptly to wash away the dead skin cells and impurities.
- Tip: alternating temperatures in the shower from hot to cold will further invigorate the skin and stimulate blood circulation, bringing more blood to the outer layers of the skin.
- Follow up by applying coconut oil to nourish the skin.

Do this for at least 30 days, just as many of the other cleanses, or make it part of your daily routine on an ongoing basis. *Cleanse your skin.*

All of the cleanses described above can be done together, and you will finish them in one month's time. If you feel you have deeper need, you may continue the cleansing phase for as long as 90 days, and during a detox, as well. Make sure to drink plenty of water and getting adequate rest to help your body with the hard work of cleansing. It's good to repeat these cleanses for 30 days at least once a year. Remember that you are taking direct steps to cleanse your organs of elimination to prepare them for the hard work of healing yourself.

Action steps:

- Cleanse the colon
- Cleanse the liver
- Cleanse the kidneys
- Cleanse the lungs
- Cleanse the skin

Additional Cleansing Techniques

Oil Pulling

Oil pulling is an ancient Ayurvedic technique of pulling toxins from the body by swishing around natural oils, such as olive or coconut, in the mouth. The added effects include teeth whitening and improved gum health, while killing localized bacteria in the mouth.

To do oil pulling, first thing in the morning, before eating or drinking, take up to one tablespoon of oil, and swish it in the mouth for 10-20 minutes. It may take a few days to work up to that length of time. Also, I can tell you from experience that you will want to have a hand towel close by in case you sneeze! Do oil pulling at least once daily, on an empty stomach, followed by brushing your teeth. Once you spit the oil out, it will look cloudy because of the toxins leached from your body. The practice is purported to provide some pretty hefty overall results, and several books have been written on oil pulling alone. Give it a try and see if it's for you!

(A note: spit the oil into a container to prevent clogging of your pipes.)

Bonus Step:

- Add Oil Pulling to your routine.

Massage

It is hard for me to over-stress the value of massage. I believe it's so beneficial that we offer massage services at our wellness center. Getting regular massages potentially can do the following for you:

- Decrease anxiety.
- Enhance sleep quality.
- Increase energy.
- Improve concentration.
- Reduce fatigue.
- Alleviate low-back pain and improve range of motion.
- Assist with shorter, easier labor for expectant mothers, and shorten maternity hospital stays.
- Ease medication dependence.

- Enhance immunity by stimulating lymph flow - the body's natural defense system.
- Exercise and stretch weak, tight, or atrophied muscles.
- Relax and soften injured, tired, and overused muscles.
- Help athletes of any level prepare for, and recover from, strenuous workouts.
- Improve the condition of the body's largest organ - the skin.
- Increase joint flexibility.
- Lessen depression and anxiety.
- Promote tissue regeneration, reducing scar tissue and stretch marks.
- Pump oxygen and nutrients into tissues and vital organs, improving circulation.
- Reduce post surgery adhesions and swelling.
- Reduce spasms and cramping.
- Release endorphins - amino acids that work as the body's natural painkillers.
- Relieve migraine pain.
- Arthritis sufferers note fewer aches, and less stiffness and pain.
- Asthmatic children show better pulmonary function and increased peak air flow.
- Burn injury patients report reduced pain, itching, and anxiety.
- High blood pressure patients demonstrate lower diastolic blood pressure, anxiety, and stress hormones.
- Premenstrual syndrome sufferers have decreased water retention and cramping.
- Preterm infants have improved weight gain.

You see, everyone benefits from massage; it's not just for pampering, although it does bring a level of "Ahhh!!!" that few other things can. If you can work it into your budget, I recommend a weekly massage, or as frequently as possible. It's sure to heighten your immune system, your energy level, and your overall sense of vitality!

Bonus Step:

- Add regular massage to your routine.

Infrared Sauna

This is another service we provide at our wellness center because I deeply believe in its benefits. Make sure you use a sauna that is of high quality, and shielded from EMFs and EMRs. (If you aren't sure what those are, you can add it to your study list!) Here are some of the benefits possible from infrared sauna.

- Detoxification: Sweating is the body's safe and natural way to heal and stay healthy, and something that we don't do nearly enough! Heating the body directly, from infrared heat, causes a rise in core temperature resulting in a deep, detoxifying sweat at the cellular level, which releases toxins.

- Relaxation: Infrared is a gentle, soothing, and therapeutic heat that promotes relaxation and improved sleep, unlike traditional saunas which operate at extremely harsh temperatures. Infrared sauna therapy helps you relax while inducing an invigorating, deep-tissue sweat. This leaves you refreshed after each session.

- Lower Blood Pressure: By inducing a deep sweat, infrared saunas make the heart pump faster. Sweating increases blood flow, lowers blood pressure, and helps circulation.

- Anti-Aging and Skin Purification: Used in spas and cosmetic centers, the near-infrared wavelength is the most effective wavelength for healing the epidermis and dermis layers of the skin. Near-infrared waves stimulate collagen production to reduce wrinkles and improve overall skin tone, enhancing a youthful appearance.

- Cell Health: Near-infrared therapy increases circulation and more fully oxygenates the body's cells. Better blood circulation improves cellular health, aids in muscle recovery, and supports the immune system.

- Weight Loss: Studies have shown that a 30-minute infrared sauna session can burn upwards of 700 calories. And this is done while you relax! By simply enjoying the sauna, there is a substantial increase in heart rate, cardiac output, and metabolic rate, which causes the body to burn more calories.

- Pain Relief: Infrared heat penetrates tissue, joints, and muscles to relieve anything from minor aches and pains to chronic pain conditions such as fibromyalgia. Healthcare professionals are using infrared heat to decrease pain and muscle spasms, and to speed up recovery time.

- Improved Circulation: Heating the muscles with infrared rays produces an increase in blood flow similar to that seen during exercise. The biggest results are gained with regular infrared sauna use. Two to three times a week will improve overall health and cardiac stamina.

- Wound Healing: Near-infrared therapy greatly enhances the skin's healing process by promoting faster cell regeneration and human tissue growth. The use of infrared sauna (especially with LED therapy) will reduce acne, and benefit most skin conditions.

I have never been someone who sweats very easily, and I know that sweating helps a person to be healthy. An old saying that has stuck with me is, "Laugh, cry, and sweat every day for good health." I'm not sure I like the cry part, but I do get it. When I took my first sauna, I was shocked to see that even my kneecaps could sweat! You can think of sweating as washing your body from the inside out. So, if you have an aversion to sweating, get over it!

Two to three sessions a week will provide the greatest benefits. It's best to start at lower temperatures, and work your way up to higher numbers. The temperature might be as low as 95, if a person is very sick, and as high as 145, if that feels like it isn't too taxing. The good thing to remember here is that all you need to do is sweat. Hotter does not equal better. My favorite temperature is between 115 and 120. The same approach should be applied to the duration of your session. I have found that the sicker someone is, lower heat for a shorter duration is best. Despite the fact that you are just sitting, your body is working, and we want to respect the strength you have available to you. Regardless of the temperature and duration of your sauna session, be sure to drink extra water and get adequate rest both prior to and after your sauna. (Contact me if you would like to know the brand of sauna that we carry in our center).

Bonus Step:

- Add infrared sauna to your routine.

Ionic Foot Detox

This modality is a very effective and quick way to pull toxins from the body. However, a good ionic foot detox system isn't readily available in every town, and to buy one that isn't a piece of junk will cost you more than a thousand dollars. Search for someone offering sessions, and then make sure their unit doesn't use POSITIVE IONS. The unit should only use NEGATIVE IONS – the ions that are good for us (counter intuitive, I know).

The ionic detox foot bath process creates a type of osmosis condition, where the negative ions are absorbed by the body through the feet. This causes toxins to be eliminated from the body, both during the session itself, and through the body's natural elimination systems for a few days after the session. At the beginning of the session, when you place your feet into the water and activate the machine, the water is clear. By the end of the session, the water has changed in color, partially due to the cellular waste and impurities that have been pulled from your body. This process of drawing impurities from the body improves the body's natural resilience. Cells photographed under a dark field microscope demonstrate marked improvements after just one bath. In these images, you can see that the cells are free-floating and rounded, appearing much more hydrated and oxygenated than they did prior to the bath. In addition, the cell walls are clearer and less dense. The technology works with the water in your body, activating it, and energizing and balancing your own body's systems.

If you try a session, and feel it is right for you, you may want to purchase a unit for yourself so you can make this detox part of your regular regimen. (Again, you can contact me for brands.)

Bonus Step:

- Add Ionic Foot Detox to your routine.

Essential Oils

These are not so much a cleansing technique as they are a health aid. Essential oils are a safe and natural way to help with symptoms of illness, and simply increase vitality and health. They are a great way to heal yourself and support your body in doing what it already wants to do: be well.

We use the oils from Young Living, but there are at least a couple of other good companies making quality essential oils. This comes right from the Young Living website:

> *Primarily extracted through careful steam distillation, but also through cold pressing, the purest essential oils are far more powerful and effective than dry herbs, delivering quick and effective results. Any time you hold a bottle of our powerful essential oils, you are holding the pure essence of health-promoting botanicals that can be diffused, inhaled, applied topically, incorporated into massage, or taken internally.*

Our family uses oils to combat or prevent common viruses, seasonal allergies, and more. You will find them an easy aid if you choose to utilize them.

Bonus Step:

- Add essential oils to your routine.

Diet

This is a touchy subject for many people; I get that. The word, alone, has connotations of self-deprivation, and of being temporary. We may even conjure up feelings of self-loathing or failure at the mere mention of the word. But I am going to challenge you to the idea that we literally "are what we eat."

While I am not a dietitian or a nutritionist, I can lend you my own experience of sorting through ill health and using food as medicine. I can offer you advice based on my own experience, and then I recommend you work with a qualified practitioner to sort out your body's needs.

In my 20s, a book came out called "Eat Right For Your Type," by naturopathic doctor Peter J. D'Adamo, N.D. As I was beginning to need to learn how to eat for good health, I was intrigued. With an A blood type, Dr. D'Adamo recommended that I eat vegetarian. I did this for awhile, felt worse, and quit. It wasn't until many years later that I realized I had eaten much more wheat when I quit eating meat. I since have discovered that I am severely allergic to gluten, so it only made sense that I would feel worse and not better when I changed my diet! After eliminating gluten from my diet, I made the switch to become vegetarian. Lo and behold, I felt MUCH BETTER! I think Dr. D'Adamo's theory makes a lot of sense, and for many people I know, changing their diet according to blood type as outlined in Dr. D'Adamo's book has brought them greater health. I recommend you read it, and see if eating the diet outlined for your blood type makes a difference for you.

Now, before we get deeply into the diet, I want to suggest that you get a food panel done. Go to the trouble of testing to determine your sensitivities and allergies. You will never get the results you want until you do this. If you are sick, you most likely have at least one hidden food sensitivity or allergy, and it is possible you have more than one. You can get this testing done through an independent lab, your own doctor, or a trained acupuncturist. People often say to me, "OH, I am FINE eating (fill in the blank). I've eaten it all my life." I have to ask them how they know whether or not they are "fine," unless they have gone 30 days without eating it. Find out what you are eating that is offending you. Your body will love you for it, and you will be well on your way to healing yourself.

From what I remember of my diet in childhood, it was nowhere near to my diet now. Thankfully, the last several years have brought a heightened awareness of, and pro-activity regarding, how and what we, as a culture, eat. With a very hardworking single father, I really didn't have a clue how to eat right. In high school, my lunches mainly consisted of donuts, soda, fries, pizza, and, if I was feeling healthy, then maybe a white bagel with cream cheese. Stacked up on top of my genetics, that type of diet was the beginning of a downward spiral in my health!

It was pregnancy that opened my eyes to the importance of what I eat. I was 18 with my first child, and suddenly, I valued the quality of the food that I ate. My resources for learning were limited, and I was being inundated with the USDA food pyramid, thanks to the Women Infants Children program. The WIC program is a great resource for families, and I deeply value their help in learning how to feed my family. The USDA officials said the old Food Pyramid, which was first used in 1992, "was overly complicated and probably was ineffective as obesity rates in the United States have soared." The old food pyramid has been replaced by the MyPlate graphic in recognition of the growing incidence of obesity in the U.S. and as of June 2, 2011, the USDA stopping using the Food Pyramid. As a USDA organization, WIC also began using the MyPlate graphic in 2011, although they didn't adopt final changes to their food packages until February 28, 2014. The food program now provides greater access to fresh fruits and vegetables, low-fat dairy including yogurt, and "whole grains."

In the last 22 years, I have done much work in learning how to eat, and more importantly, how to use food as medicine. I firmly believe that with every bite we take, *we are either fueling disease, or healing it.*

In short, the problem with the American diet is that it is full of processed and dead foods. These foods are missing vital elements that heal and nurture the body. Furthermore, these dead foods fill us with empty calories so we are both overweight and malnourished. Junk foods cause inflammation in our bodies, which is a leading root of disease. To boot, we leave out essential elements because we have been lied to and told that they are bad for us. While most of us do the best we can with what we know, our poor dietary choices start at birth (and some would say before).

In The Beginning

Many of us were not breastfed (I thank GOD that I was!), or if we were, it was not for very long. The average age of weaning in the U.S. is three months. In contrast, the average age for weaning worldwide is 4.2 years. The World Health Organization claims that breastfeeding should continue for at least two years. Interestingly, two years is the average age for the immune system's maturation. In addition, the American

Academy of Pediatrics recommends breastfeeding for at least one year.
It seems most parents believe that once baby is eating a well-rounded diet of solids, breast milk is no longer important.

When it comes to breast milk, there is no more nutritionally-dense food available to a human. Studies have shown that breastfed children over 12 months old take in much more energy and nutrients than non-breastfed babies. Studies also have proven that children who are breastfed have higher IQs, and the duration of breastfeeding impacts the score on the IQ tests. The disease-protective factors in breast milk become more concentrated as the child grows older. Studies show that many of the immune-boosting benefits of breastfeeding are lifelong.

You may be asking, "Why are we talking about breastfeeding here?" Well, it matters! It matters to your own state of health, and even though we can't change the past, we can impact the health of future generations, either ourselves, or through others.

I have four children of my own, and then I was a gestational surrogate. This means I carried someone else's baby to term, and gave birth to her for them. Once she was born, I nursed her for a month, and then continued to pump milk and ship it to her in another country for three more months. The loving parents were dedicated and committed to providing her with the best health possible throughout her life. We were able to supply her with breast milk for her first six months of life. While this isn't very long, it is a great accomplishment for a baby born to someone other than her mother. I'll never forget sitting in a hot tub a couple of months after she was born, and having a conversation with a NICU nurse. This nurse commended me, when she told me, "You have literally changed the health status of her 80s and 90s." While I knew how important it was to do this for my surrogate baby, hearing it from a woman who deals with breastfeeding first hand was very affirming. So, even though this has nothing to do with healing yourself, whenever you have the ability to impact a mother and child, encourage prolonged breastfeeding.

This may flip some readers out, but consider it bonus information. Some very ill adults have supplemented their diet with breast milk and had amazing results. If you have a lactating mom in your life who's willing to help, and you are sufficiently motivated to regain your health, this may be something to consider.

Going Against the Grain

You don't have to believe in cavemen to understand the idea behind the caveman diet, a/k/a the Paleo Diet. The idea is that if something has to be processed, it is not an ideal food to consume. To further the understanding, the diet is based on the assumption that humans are hunter-gatherers, and if something cannot be hunted or gathered, then it can cause the breakdown of our bodies; i.e., disease.

As hunter-gatherers, humans historically ate foods such as seafood (fish, mammals, shellfish, seaweed); land mammals (including organs, fat, and marrow); vegetables (stems, leaves, etc.); cooked tubers; fruit; eggs; nuts; honey; mushrooms; birds; and insects. How much we ate, and of what, varied from group to group, but this was the general diet of hunter-gatherers, and is thought to be pretty much what we've been living on for the last 1.5 million years or so. The Paleo Diet would have us continue to eat this type of fresh-food diet, avoiding all processed foods.

Now, you may be arguing with me or balking at the idea of eating like this. But, honestly tell me, don't you know somewhere inside that cookies aren't good for us? I mean, are chips good for us? What about donuts? Soda? Okay, but what about crackers and bread? PASTA, FOR GOD'S SAKE? I mean, we need those to get vital nutrients for our bodies, right? What about all those so-called "whole grain" breads? Those are good for us, right? And, you may be saying, "My morning cereal is all natural granola. THAT has got to be good for me!"

NOPE, NOPE, and sorry, but NO.

Science, through archeology, is showing that as grains were introduced to a group of people, their bodies were impacted to their detriment. As a population began eating grains, its members began to show tooth decay, reduced stature, and reduced bone density, as well as a higher incidence of deformations and disease.

And when I say grain, I mean *every* grain. If a food must be processed (altered), then it is not natural to the body, and is therefore taxing it. You likely have heard that wheat has become a bad guy, and rightly so, but all grains must be processed to be consumed. Imagine that you are stranded somewhere on land with no one or nothing around. Hunger was driving you to search for food, and you found a rice patty, or a wheat field. Just imagine standing there looking at this crop. Go ahead, eat it. You can't, can you? You could take all day long, but you could not gather enough grain to make much of an impact on your nutritional needs. In addition, you would need a pot and water to process it over fire. Now, imagine that you are walking and you find your favorite fruit tree. Reach up, and pick it. Go ahead, eat it. When you are finished, continue walking until you find leafy greens, vegetables of any sort, and maybe some nuts. Craving some meat? Well, you will have to devise a weapon of some sort, but that is an option. Many cultures eat it raw, but using fire to cook it isn't out of the question. Cooking meat simply reduces the risk of disease. Eating raw meat is completely an option, physically. (Nevertheless, I do not recommend that you eat raw meat in any situation unless you are trained to do so).

Are you getting the picture now? Grains cause inflammation and do horrible things to our body, either directly or indirectly. Almost all plant food contains some kind of toxin, but grains produce quite a few nasty ones that can do harm. Grains contain a large amount of phytic acid, for example. The phytic acid significantly inhibits our absorption of many important minerals. When a group of people adopt grains as their carbohydrate-rich food in place of tubers, they are taking on a load of toxins and giving up a lot of nutrients that their bodies need. Tubers were our main carbohydrate source for the 1.5 million years before agriculture, and tubers contain far less phytic acid than grains. There are a number of other toxins that occur in grains but not in tubers, such as certain heat-resistant lectins. In addition to these toxins, common to all grain is a substance called gluten, which is a compound of two proteins. Gluten creates reactions in everyone's body, ranging from mild to traumatic. All of these reasons likely explain why stature decreased when humans began consuming grain. With modern farming and processing methods, the gluten in wheat has increased dramatically, causing wheat and gluten sensitivity and allergy to become one of our fastest rising afflictions.

I feel a bit aggravated when I read claims that gluten is found only in wheat, barley, and rye. That isn't true. There is gluten in every single grain. Yes, the incredible manipulation and sometimes genetic modification of wheat, barley, and rye have bastardized those grains into "super enemies," but every grain has the potential to cause this harm. Don't forget that corn is a grain, as well. The type of gluten and name of it changes, but it exists in every grain, and has the potential to create inflammation and reduce the efficacy of nutrient absorption. One of the basic ways grains reduce nutrient absorption is their creation of a glue-like coating on the intestinal wall, thereby limiting intake of nutrients from the food passing through. Another way gluten causes problems is that it acts as an irritant, causing inflammation in the lining of the intestines. In many people, this inflammation eventually causes leaks in the intestinal walls, letting the food particles pass into the abdominal cavity. When this happens, the body's immune system reacts to that food particle as an enemy. This condition is called leaky gut syndrome. The whole immune army is then on the lookout for this enemy, and the body develops various symptoms as a result of consuming the offender. When this scenario continues long enough, the body starts attacking anything that looks like the enemy. This is the case in gluten ataxia and celiac disease. Doctors are beginning to suspect many more disorders are related to this scenario, as well.

Much of my learning about food as medicine was by default and need. When my third child, my first daughter, was born, she was colicky, and my midwife told me that 95% of the time, cutting out dairy will stop it. I did, and it worked. Then, this baby also began developing eczema, and I, again, asked my midwife. She informed me that the most common cause of eczema is wheat. I cut it out of my diet, and lo and behold, my daughter's eczema cleared up. I was beginning to gain a deep appreciation for food as medicine.

When my next child, also a daughter, was born, she also was colicky, and I again quit eating dairy. She cheered right up. Then, I noticed she had a stuffy nose all the time and seemed to have difficulty breathing. I again cut out the wheat, and she could breathe clearly!

When the surrogate baby was born, she, too, was a bit colicky, and I cut out the dairy. Two years later, when my health was at its lowest, I went back on my wheat-free, dairy-free diet, because I recalled feeling my best when I was nursing my daughters. Almost magically, many of the symptoms I was experiencing disappeared. I no longer had digestive issues like before. I had energy and wasn't overcome with exhaustion. The fog of depression lifted, and I had fewer aches and pains.

As I investigated and talked to doctors, I found that few of them had an appreciation for the toxicity of foods, and some actually told me that if I were healthy, my body would tolerate any food. Well, that is a FAST way to anger a patient with obvious food sensitivities/allergies. I'm sure you can imagine that living for a year with the knowledge that I was seriously allergic to gluten, but not having any doctor acknowledge the depth of this, was strenuous, to say the least. Some friends and family members were less than supportive of my 'self-diagnosis.' Imagine my relief when the top specialist I was sent to agreed that my disease was most likely from Gluten. I felt great comfort and validation in being taken seriously.

You may be thinking, "I can't LIVE without my grains!" Guess what? You actually may be *addicted* to gluten! As gluten is digested, it forms gluten exorphins – opioid peptides that can bind to receptors in the brain, disrupting brain function. Thus, eating gluten may actually give you a "high," making you feel good, happy, and just plain . . . "Yeah, man."

After spending much time studying grains and their effects on the body, I have concluded that, sadly, they are quite the enemy. I only allow myself to consume a couple of servings of organic, whole-grain rice or corn each week. I also should mention that I am primarily vegan, but sometimes, I need more than fruits, vegetables, nuts, and seeds!

By now, you may be thinking this section is a plug for the Paleo Diet. YEP. You've got that right. It is time that we get back to our natural diet. It is time that we consume food whose waste is bones, peels, pits, and skins, instead of wrappers and boxes. YES, I am passionate about this! Gluten from grains has attacked my brain and nervous system, and it has attacked my children's bodies. Can you blame me for my passion?

I recommend you read The Grain Brain by David Perlmutter, M.D., and challenge your attachment to grains. Another good read is Wheat Belly by William Davis, M.D.

If you look at the USDA Food Pyramid, or follow their current info graph that they are using, you will see their recommendation for grains is ½ - ¼ of your food should come from grains! If you consider all the information I have shared with you so far, you will see the USDA is recommending that ONE FOURTH of your daily food intake be from food that will do you harm! In my view, that recommendation is irresponsible, and actually akin to a death sentence for many people. I further believe that recommendation is a leading reason that when you go out in public, you will see that a growing percentage of our population is obese and sick. We are sick and we are fat, and it is because we are overfed and undernourished. We feed on grains like we are cows (even though cows also shouldn't be grain fed). I can't help but notice the connection; we line up to be served these portions of dead grains, and find ourselves fattening up and developing disease.

How did we ever get to the place where our government is telling us we should be taking half of our food from grains? That came about as more and more farms were being subsidized for growing grains, which are very profitable crops. To produce a bowl of cereal as compared to a steak is a huge financial difference, and not just for the consumer. Farms produce grain because that is what has been encouraged, and producers promote grain consumption because the product needs to be moved. So, advertisers convince us that grains are an essential component to a healthy heart, waistline, or whatever else moves us to consume it.

At some point, we have to wake up, step up, and take charge of the food that goes into our mouths. We have to make a decision to go against the grain (pun intended), and change the state of our health. I also suggest you take one hour, and watch a documentary called [Cereal Killers](), by D.J. O'Neill. The documentary blows open the idea of the USDA Food Pyramid, and does so brilliantly. You ARE what you eat. If you want to be alive and full of energy, you must eat food that is such!

What Fuels Disease

Inflammation is being identified as the source of many diseases. If you have suffered from pain, obesity, ADD/ADHD, peripheral neuropathy, diabetes, heart disease, stroke, migraines, thyroid issues, dental issues, or cancer, you are suffering from inflammation. In order to heal from these and any other diseases, we must get rid of the inflammation.

Our gut is the primary source of inflammation, and the semi-permeable lining is the vulnerable target. When stretched out flat, the surface area of our intestinal lining would cover two tennis courts! Unfortunately, this semi-permeable lining fluctuates with respect to how permeable it is. You may be shocked to know that the intestinal wall is only ONE CELL THICK! When our cortisol levels are high, due to stress, or our thyroid function is strained, the intestinal lining becomes more permeable. What does this mean for us? Well, when we eat, partially-undigested food, toxins, viruses, yeast, and bacteria can pass through this lining and enter the bloodstream. This is called leaky gut syndrome. When this condition is repeated again and again, inflammation occurs, and often, along with it, allergic reactions to the food that you eat.

Smoldering inflammation is so common in our bodies that it can go on for years before it becomes apparent. By that point, we often are fighting disease. In addition to inflammation in the gut, chronic inflammation can reside in the joints and the tissues of the body. Chronic inflammation is associated with the most deadly diseases that we face.

Eating properly and making appropriate lifestyle choices are our approaches to reducing and preventing inflammation. Smoking, drinking alcohol, and eating junk food are the fastest ways to create this inflammation. Knowing that inflammation is within our control should be encouraging!

What are the foods that cause inflammation?

- SUGAR – all sweets and sugars. Sugar is one of the most addictive substances that we consume. According to the USDA, each American consumes 156 pounds of various sources of sugars a year via candy, cookies, sodas, juices, and various treats. Through a series of chemical changes that occur when we consume sugar, inflammation sets in. Is it any wonder that our highly sweet diets lead to disease?

- PROCESSED, PACKAGED, OR PREPARED – Fast food is full of harmful oils, sugar and artificial sweeteners, food additives, and a lot more harmful chemicals.

- HYDROGENATED AND TRANS FATS – These are the fats found in shortening, margarine, and lard. Cooking oils containing these fats are used in most baked goods and sweets.

- MEAT – As you know by now, I am a fan of the Paleo diet, so although I've included meat in this list, I caution that you should not reduce your meat consumption if you find you are not sensitive to meat. For most people, it isn't the meat that causes inflammation; it's the harmful chemicals within the meat due to the way the animals are treated. They are injected with hormones and other chemicals, and fed pesticide-laden grains. In addition, their bodies may excrete extreme amounts of stress hormones due to the cruelty of their living conditions. If you are going to eat meat, eat clean, humanely-raised, organic meat. Yes, it costs more, but you are worth it.

- FOOD ADDITIVES – From flavor enhancers, preservatives, stabilizers, and artificial coloring, we are eating a veritable chemistry experiment. If a substance doesn't occur naturally, it shouldn't go into or onto our bodies.

- FRIED FOODS – We go back to the bad fats now. All of our favorite comfort foods that are deep-fried are laden with bad fats. Those French-fries, potato chips, and fried chicken just aren't going to serve you in your quest to maintain good health, no matter how you dress them.

- SYNTHETIC SWEETENERS – Any sweetener that isn't naturally-occurring has many more harmful effects than natural sweeteners. Just DON'T put them in your body.

- DAIRY PRODUCTS – Most dairy products you will get your hands on are laden with hormones, antibiotics, and other additives. Unless you buy organic, 100% natural dairy products, just avoid them. If you ARE consuming them, keep it to no more than one serving a day. Now, an added bit of information is that cow's milk is very different from human milk. If you are inclined to consume dairy, I highly recommend going to goat's or sheep's milk/cheeses, which resemble human milk much more closely, and are much kinder to the body. Although I am primarily vegan, I do indulge in some goat/sheep cheese.

- WHEAT – Wheat is very acid-forming and causes inflammation in the body. If you must consume wheat, consume it rarely, and make sure it is organic, non-GMO, and ancient grain.

- GLUTEN – Gluten is found in EVERY grain. That means rice, oats, and corn as well as the wheat, kamut, barley, and rye. Grains are processed. They have to be, as they are inedible without being processed. Corn is one of the most highly genetically-modified foods that we eat, and it seems to be in almost everything. I don't like it any more than you do, but the fact is, we have to quit eating it. So, again, if you can't hunt it or gather it, it really isn't going to do your body any good. Gluten, itself, is the cause of many of the health problems we face, and we will be much healthier if we avoid it altogether.

- ALCOHOL – All alcohol turns to sugar in our bodies, so it is no different than eating sugar. Sure, tipping a glass of red wine seems much more refined than licking a lollipop, but it really isn't. Alcohol burdens the liver, as well, and it is best to reduce this and consider what you are really putting into your body. Yes, there are some studies claiming to prove some health benefits from drinking moderate portions of red wine. I won't take that from you because I, too, like red wine. The rule of thumb, in consuming wine or anything else, is moderation.

By eliminating or reducing the inflammatory foods we consume, we can make an immediate impact on our overall health. This is why so many people have great results when they go on a healthy diet that eliminates the previously-mentioned foods.

What Heals Disease

In addition to eliminating inflammatory foods, you should eat lots of fresh vegetables and fruits (three times more vegetables than fruits). Make sure you are getting at least two cups of green, leafy vegetables every day. Adding RAW nuts and seeds to your daily diet will help you immensely, and I recommend soaking/sprouting for the best results (you can only do this with raw nuts). Un-soaked/sprouted nuts and seeds contain enzymes that prevent them from being broken down. These enzymes can make it hard for them to be digested fully, and even cause gas and bloating. By soaking/sprouting your nuts and seeds, you are releasing healthy components that otherwise wouldn't be available for your body to utilize.

Also add lots of clean, "living" water to your routine. Most of us walk around dehydrated, and are completely accustomed to it. Daily, you should drink half your body weight in ounces (e.g., if you weigh 150 pounds, you should 75 ounces of water). Make sure you are using a high-quality water filtration device that also adds minerals back into the water. We use the water system from Nikken.

Eat enough fat! If you took time to study the Paleo diet, you know your diet should include healthy fats. The majority of people don't eat enough healthy fat, and that is why we are obese and sick. As a vegan, it is difficult for me to get enough fat, so I eat plenty of nuts, seeds, and olives, as well as a fair amount of avocados). If you are not vegetarian or vegan, your choices for fat are greater. Don't trim the fat off of the meat. Eat it, and let your body more easily digest the meat, as well as enjoy feeling satisfied longer.

Cut out the bedtime snack. Your body does not need fuel to sleep. It needs to utilize its energy to repair and restore the body, not to digest. Eating before bed can cause disturbed sleep. Finish eating at dinnertime, and let your body enjoy a true nighttime fast.

If certain foods cause inflammation, are there foods that reduce inflammation? I'm so glad that you asked that question! There are many foods that will give you a boost in fighting inflammation, and I will list them here.

- GOOD OILS – Oils that contain oleic acid (an omega-9 fatty acid) such as olive, grape seed, and avocado oils. These are especially good for your heart and brain.

- FISH – For those of you who are not vegetarian or vegan, fish is a great anti-inflammatory food. Fish is high in omega-3 fatty acid. Vegan sources are nuts, seeds, and seaweed.

- NUTS AND FRUITS – These foods are a great natural weapon against inflammation. The nuts and seeds are best if they are raw and sprouted.

- GARLIC – As a woman married to a Greek, I can say this one is our favorites! It tastes good (and if you don't like it, you will get used to it). It helps to reduce swollen joints, as well, and combat an array of other issues.

- HERBS – The fresher, the better. Basil, oregano, parsley, rosemary, chili peppers (be careful with these for inflammation in the gut), thyme, ginger, and turmeric all fight inflammation.

- CHOCOLATE – Yes, this seems to go against the whole recommendation not to eat sweets, but a healthy chocolate has little sugar in it. Choose at least 70% cocoa, and you will have a tasty way to combat disease. (Did I mention moderation in all things?)

- GREEN TEA – This will reduce the risk of heart disease, and is anti-inflammatory and loaded with antioxidants. If you are sensitive to caffeine (like me), then try non-caffeinated herbal teas for much of the same benefit.

By changing the way you eat, you will change each and every cell in your body. Good food can renew you and make you stronger.

It's taken me years to be at a place with food that I feel both confident and healthy. Currently, I am vegan, other than a meat indulgence once a week if I am deeply craving meat. I also am mostly grain free, with a once or twice a week indulgence of an organic, non-GMO grain (usually rice or quinoa). I allow myself to have a few servings of sheep/goat feta each week. I eat mostly vegetables all day, with a couple servings of fruit. For fat, I consume avocados, olive oil, nuts, seeds, and coconut, and little bit of feta. It has taken me a couple of years to refine and sort out my diet. I feel healthy and strong, and listen to my body. I now know when I have eaten something that my body is sensitive or allergic to. If I feel a deep need for a certain clean, healthy food, then I will eat it. I now eat out of an understanding of what the food is, and how it can serve me, and I have a healthy dose of respect for how it can impact my health.

Having leaky gut syndrome has been challenging, in that there have been many foods I am sensitive or allergic to. However, I've been patient with myself, and understand that, in time, changing my diet has been healing. As an added benefit, I now am able to tolerate some foods that I wasn't able to before. It can feel very challenging to know how and what your body wants you to feed it, but the payoff is enormous. By ridding your diet of the offending foods and adding in healing foods, you will heal yourself in ways that nothing else could.

Supplementation

Modern intensive agricultural methods have stripped increasing amounts of nutrients from the soil in which the food we eat grows. You just can't get enough nutrition from the food you eat today due to soil depletion and over-farming. America has the highest rates of soil depletion, as compared to any other nation. How does this happen? Farmers grow crops, taking essential nutrients out of the soil. Then they stick another crop in over and over again, with little rest for the land or replacement of the lost minerals. In addition to the pulling of the nutrients out of the soil, the food products themselves have been bred and manipulated so they are increasingly bigger, and more pest resistant, with little focus on increasing their nutritional impact.

The state of American health shows that we are over-fed and malnourished. For anyone dealing with an illness, supplementation will be a great advantage in the healing process. Note, however, that the choices and possibilities available for supplementation of vitamins and minerals is staggering. I don't suggest you undertake this on your own, but get a trained person to guide you. This could be an acupuncturist, a nutritionist, or a naturopath.

I suggest you get tested for any deficiencies, and let that be the starting place for your selection of supplements. Depending on which professional you choose, they may suggest a blood panel or other methods of detecting your deficiencies.

Action Steps:

- Choose someone to guide you through nutritional supplementation.
- Take your supplements faithfully.

Output

So, we have talked about what goes into our mouths. Let's talk about the other end. Many of us were taught, growing up, not to talk about what people do in the bathroom. No one wants to know about that! Sadly, the result is that most people don't have any idea of what constitutes a healthy bowel movement. Children grow up constipated because no one talks to them about their bathroom habits, and adults live with constipation, not knowing this is one of the reasons they are sick.

Well, I am ready to get "down and dirty" with you here about poop. It wasn't until my 30s that I learned how I should be pooping – and not just me, but you, too. Come to find out, I had been constipated all of my life. If you are not having two to three bowel movements a day that come without strain or splashing into the water, then you are constipated. Your food should not take more than 24 hours to clear your body. If it does, is it any wonder you don't feel great with putrefying food sitting in your gut? Your specimen should hold together, and be about the length of your forearm (notice I said length, and not size). Nope, I'm not kidding. There are many healthy people who can do this several times a day.

Thankfully, just by changing your diet, you are well on your way. And knowing what your bowel movements should be like is a great tool in assessing whether or not a certain food is offensive to your body. If your bowel movements change, all you have to do is look at the food you are eating to identify why.

How do you have bowel movements 2-3 times a day of this caliber?
1. Drink half your bodyweight in ounces of water each day (e.g., if you weigh 150 pounds, drink 75 ounces of water).
2. Eat lots of vegetables, including leafy greens, daily.
3. Quit eating grains.
4. Quit eating or reduce dairy.
5. Eliminate all food to which you are allergic/sensitive.

You can find more information on having healthy bowel movements all over the internet. Knowing what you should be experiencing is the first step to developing healthy habits.

Action Steps:

- Get tested for food sensitivities/allergies.
- Get tested for deficiencies and begin supplementation.
- Eliminate offending foods and add healing foods.
- Drink half your body weight in ounces of water a day.

Sound Therapy

You don't have to have a condition of the brain to appreciate Sound Therapy. As a person with compromises of the brain that are part of my diseases, I deeply value sound therapy, and implement it into my life. Basically, to understand sound therapy, you have to appreciate that everything in life has a vibration. Every living and unliving thing has a vibration to it, and these vibrations have different frequencies. The frequencies have an effect on how we feel.

If you aren't sure that sound and vibration have an effect on us, think back to a time when you were deeply enjoying some of your favorite music. You probably actually *felt* different in some way. Maybe you were moved emotionally. Maybe you just couldn't help moving your body to the rhythm. Similarly, think of how you feel when you sing, or chant. Your whole body is affected. Sound vibrations make an impact on our physical body and our state of mind.

Our brain waves play a deeply impactful role in the effects of the vibrations that flood our body. First of all, let's understand brain waves.

- Gamma – 27 Hz and up – Gamma is associated with the formation of ideas, language, and memory processing, and various types of learning. Gamma waves have been shown to disappear during deep sleep induced by anesthesia, but return with the transition back to a wakeful state.

- Beta – 12hz to 27 hz – Wide awake. This is generally the mental state most people are in during the day and most of their waking lives. Usually, this state, in and of itself, is uneventful, but don't underestimate its importance. Many people lack sufficient beta activity, which can cause mental or emotional disorders such as depression, ADD, and insomnia.

- Alpha – 8 hz to 12 hz – Awake, but relaxed and not processing much information. When you get up in the morning, and just before sleep, you are naturally in this state. When you close your eyes, your brain automatically starts producing more alpha waves. Alpha activity has also been connected to the ability to recall memories, lessened discomfort and pain, and reductions in stress and anxiety.

- Theta – 3 hz to 8 hz – Light sleep or extreme relaxation. Theta is also a very receptive mental state that has proven useful for hypnotherapy, as well as self-hypnosis using recorded affirmations and suggestions.

- Delta - .2 hz to 3 hz – Deep, dreamless sleep. Delta is the slowest band of brainwaves. When your dominant brainwave is delta, your body is healing itself and resetting its internal clocks. You do not dream in this state, and are completely unconscious.

Now, I will introduce you to what may be a new term to you: binaural beats. Using binaural beats is a method of using sound to essentially reset the brain waves. To listen to a binaural beat, you use headphones to bring sound to each ear. Each tone is at a slightly different frequency, which results in the beat that you perceive. You can use the above information on brain waves to begin choosing binaural beats that will suit your needs. The best time to do this is when you are resting or sleeping. For rest and sleep, you would choose alpha, delta, or theta waves. You can use beta or gamma binaural beats to feel wakeful.

If all of this information about sound therapy confuses or overwhelms you, a simple way to increase your health and vitality is to listen to classical music. Make a habit of listening to a type of classical music that suits you, and your body will thank you for it. It's not as precise as binaural beats, but it will make a difference. Research shows that listening to classical music while pregnant increases the IQ of the child. If that is so, we can extrapolate that it is good for adults, as well.

Amanda Angel, who blogs for New York Public Radio station WQXR, did a good job of pulling together information on the effects of listening to classical music in her November 10, 2011, article, "Top Five Studies on Classical Music and Health." Angel notes studies have shown that listening to classical music lowers blood pressure, relieves post-surgical pain, heightens emotions, aids sleep, lessens symptoms associated with epilepsy, and actually may make you smarter! You can read the entire article here.

So, put on that music and enjoy healing yourself while you simply live, work, and play!

Bonus Step:

- Add binaural beat and/or classical music to your routine.

Rest and Relaxation

This one is near and dear to my heart. As a born "Type A" person, resting, for me, has always come with a heavy dose of guilt and discomfort. Through the challenges I have been given, I have had to learn both the value of, and appreciation for, resting and relaxing. Quite literally, when a body is worn out, we must sit down and put our feet up. But sometimes it takes more than that. Sometimes, our bodies are so worn out from constant stress that we not only need to sit down and put our feet up, we also need to close our eyes and enjoy some of those brain waves with lower frequencies! Remember our earlier discussion about the effects of stress.

Our modern-day bodies and lives are full of stimulation and activity. Our bodies are deeply in need of rest and relaxation. If you are suffering from a disease or health challenge of any kind, you likely need more rest. (Of course, this isn't true for everyone; some of us get enough rest, or maybe even too much. We will talk about that more in the next section.)

If you are active, work, or care for a family, and find yourself feeling overly tired, then you need to give the body what it is asking for in order for it to heal. Most modern people don't value or respect the need to rest the body, but you are reading this book because you are ready to heal, right?

Napping is a common activity in many cultures, including the Mediterranean and Spanish cultures. By laying down each day for 30 to 90 minutes (hopefully, listening to some healing music), you are allowing your body to repair and heal itself. Putting your feet up at least as high as your heart gives the cardiovascular system a break.

My work schedule doesn't allow a full rest every day, but three times a week, I lie down and take a nap. In addition to that, I have learned to take short breaks at work, putting my feet up, and doing nothing 'productive,' allowing my brainwaves to change and my body to reboot.

So, love yourself, and take a rest every day, if you can work it into your schedule. In addition, get to bed no later than 10:00 or 11:00 each night. Our bodies need to be asleep by this time, and your sleep will be more effective, leaving you feeling more alert and refreshed when you awaken.

Action Step:

- Build regular rest periods into your schedule, and then take those breaks (even when you don't want to).

Exercise

Well, surely, this is *the* most dear to my heart. When I became pregnant the first time, I knew that exercising was important to be healthy, so I began walking. After the baby was born, I needed to find something to help me get the weight off, and I found classes on TV that I could exercise with. After a second child, I found Pilates and then yoga. When I found yoga, I really found my fitness "home." My body became more supple and strong, and my energy improved. That was it; I was hooked, and obviously still am.

The ancient teachings of yoga originally came from Shamanistic, Hindu, and Buddhist cultures, but yoga, itself, is a science whose aim is to allow the practitioner to create a closer existence with his/her creator in his/her own system of belief.

Everyone can practice yoga, no matter their faith. If you visit a yoga class where you see symbols or hear teachings from various religious traditions tied in with yoga instruction, it may be the teacher's intention simply to share one of many views and belief systems. Be sure to let the teacher know if his/her references to particular faith traditions make you uncomfortable.

As a yoga teacher and studio owner, my whole life is about serving both my own body, and the bodies of people in our community, with yoga. For myself, I have to practice first thing in the morning if I want to have a pain-free day. When I first began practicing yoga, I was a "lean, mean yoga machine." I could do just about anything with my body. Now, about 15 years later, that is no longer the case. I sympathize with our students who come in with arthritis, injuries, aches and pains, and limitations in their bodies.

One of the effects of dystonia in my body is that my whole right side is tightening constantly. All of the muscles and fascia on the right side of my body are tighter than those on the left. This causes great imbalance in my body, if I just let it go. I must work diligently and regularly to create balance and symmetry in my body in order to feel well and pain free. However, it does cause some pain to do the practice. In addition to the effects of dystonia, I have arthritis down my left side in my low back, hip, and neck. Nevertheless, I maintain my regular yoga practice, even though it's sometimes uncomfortable. I'm telling you this because I feel that we often shy away from exercise because it is hard or uncomfortable. An important disclaimer here is that, in general, yoga should not be painful. But if you have certain conditions, it may feel uncomfortable, and you will need an intelligent teacher to guide you.

If you are sick, you likely don't feel like exercising, but I can promise you that if you don't take up some form of healthy exercise, you will not attain the level of health you desire. In my opinion, yoga is the best form of exercise, and is suitable for everyone's body. The aim of the physical practice of yoga is to create strength where there is weakness, suppleness where there is tension, and balance where there is imbalance. As long as you have breath, you can do yoga. In general, I can't recommend that you begin with yoga classes at a gym, unless you confirm that the instructor is at least a 200-hour Registered Yoga Teacher (RYT-200) through Yoga Alliance, meaning they have taken a comprehensive teacher training on how to instruct yoga properly and safely. Instead, I recommend you go to the trouble to find a yoga studio, and get a consult to find the right class for you. Better yet, find a private instructor to meet your exact needs.

A well-matched yoga practice will leave you having more energy during the day, rather than leaving you exhausted and less energetic. I am not a fan of running or jogging, and believe they are more damaging than they are beneficial. Walking is a decent alternative. I predict that the boom of aerobic exercise soon will lose its ground. You will find that a well-rounded yoga practice will meet all of your exercise needs, and will have an even deeper impact on your mind and spirit.

If you need to practice at home, or the cost of professional instruction isn't possible, then there is nothing wrong with trying a suitable DVD. There are also many great books on the market that can guide you well.

Ideally, you will do a minimum of 10 minutes of exercise each day. A good routine would be 30-60 minutes, three to six days a week. One day of complete rest is a good recommendation for most. However, if you suffer from arthritis, taking a day off will do more harm than good, so on the seventh day, do some extremely gentle movement for just 10 minutes or so.

Now, I want to speak to those of you who are feeling very proud right now because you already exercise. In fact, you exercise every day for one to two hours. Sometimes, you do back-to-back Zumba classes! Over-exercising can be just as damaging to your body as the list of inflammatory foods that we shared previously. It can be just as bad for you as not sleeping. Over-exercising is strangely prevalent today in the American culture. It seems there are just as many people who over-exercise as there are who don't exercise at all.

When you over-exercise, you are breaking down your body, using up too much of the energy needed to keep you balanced and heal you. Go back and re-read the section on getting adequate rest. We need balance in all things. Six to nine hours of exercise per week is a good maximum. If you have been over-exercising for a long time, it would serve you well to cut back.

Again, the idea is moderation in all things, but the basic truth is: Use It or Lose It. You must use your body, or your body will break down and age rapidly.

Action Step:

- Choose an exercise regimen, set a regular schedule, and stick with it.

Alignment

They say that things happen when the stars align. There seems to be this universal truth about alignment, and it is true for our bodies, as well. Our bones, tissues, and nerves all have an appointed place in our body. When these parts are out of place, which they are often and easily, we are compromised. Our bodies are soft and pliable in nature, with on the bones, tendons, and ligaments making up the firm structure. However, the firm structures come in many parts that can move out of place.

The compromise from this movement may be subtle, or it may be staggering, depending on the severity, the length of time the misalignment has occurred, and the state of the individual's health. In any state, the alignment should be rectified in order to achieve good flow of energy, optimum circulation of vital fluids, and relief of discomfort.

If you have benefitted from chiropractic care, you already understand these things. If you have not, then it's time to learn. According to the American Chiropractic Association, the roots of chiropractic care date back "to the beginning of recorded time," showing up in writings from as long ago as 2700 B.C. The benefits of spinal manipulation are recognized in some of the most ancient texts. Chiropractic treatment can be of great value to you in your quest to be well. In fact, there are few maladies that can't be helped with this care. If you have not done so, seek out a Doctor of Chiropractic (D.C.), and see how you may benefit from this service.

In this same line of thinking are acupuncture and Chinese medicine. What chiropractic care is to the bones, acupuncture and Chinese medicine are to the body's energy. There is no greater way to align the energetic body than with acupuncture and Chinese medicine. A Doctor of Chinese Medicine (sometimes called a Doctor of Oriental Medicine, or O.M.) can guide you through your nutritional needs, as well. Consider adding this practitioner to your box of tools.

Bonus Step:

- See a chiropractor and/or a Chinese medicine doctor.

Heal Your Mind

The Power of Thoughts

My father was a preacher, and as a child, I witnessed him teach the power of the spoken word. The denominations I grew up in were faith-based, and trusted heavily on the grace and mercy of God. One of the lessons taught was that the power of the spoken word is mighty and not to taken for granted. There were many instances of people with illness or injuries being healed through prayer. Through the teachings of the Bible (and many other great works), you can learn how impactful the power of our thoughts and beliefs are.

In my 20s, I experienced a period of secondary infertility. For two years, I suffered disappointment after disappointment, and much heartbreak, as I lost two babies. After two years, something in me clicked, and I went back to these teachings from my childhood. As I opened my Bible, I found a verse that inspired me to believe I would conceive and carry a healthy baby girl to term. Daily, I meditated on and prayed over Mark 11:24, "Therefore I tell you, whatever you ask for in prayer, believe that you have received it, and it will be yours." It just so happened that we were going on vacation to Hawaii the very next month, and I claimed I would come home pregnant with a healthy baby girl. Nine months later, I gave birth to Faith Manalani (heavenly power).

Research has been done to show how people who take a placebo will achieve their desired results simply by the power of their mind. Dr. Lisa Rankin documents this fact with hard science that the mind can heal the body. She notes that patients treated with placebos don't just feel better, and it's not just "in their heads." These patients have had warts disappear, bronchi dilate, colons become less inflamed, hair growth on the heads of bald men, ulcers heal, and other measurable signs of healing. We also know the opposite is true, and the mind can make the body sick. Researchers call this the nocebo effect. Dr. Rankin says that when patients are given injections with saline, and told it is chemotherapy, they vomit and lose their hair.

We are going to delve deeper into our thinking, and how it impacts our health and our disease.

Worry

Worrying is feeling unease or being overly-concerned about a situation or problem. When you worry excessively, your mind and body go into overdrive, and you constantly focus on "what might happen." When consumed with excessive worrying, you may suffer with high anxiety or even panic attacks.

Chronic worrying is so detrimental to your health that it interferes with your appetite, lifestyle habits, relationships, sleep, and job performance. People who worry excessively are prone to harmful lifestyle habits such as overeating, cigarette smoking, or using alcohol and other drugs.

I can remember my impressions of my father worrying when I was a child. I can recall the anguish and suffering that worrying caused him, and I think I must have made a decision not to worry as an adult. Now, granted, my single father, raising three children, had a lot to worry about. Life, for any human, can provide reasons to worry, and give all of us opportunities to worry when things go wrong.

However, as we have just discussed, the power of our thoughts is stronger and more impactful than most people really appreciate. If we attract what we think about, then it works the same whether we entertain crap or happiness, right? Worrying literally changes the chemistry in the body, and sets you up to entertain a host of inflammation and disease.

Let's face it, there is no reason to continue thinking about what could go wrong. Entertaining troublesome thoughts is about as pointless as anything could be. It's valuable to consider all aspects of the situations we face, but it is much more joyful to go through life focusing on what could go RIGHT! When it gets right down to it, you can either entertain a positive thought or a negative thought; you cannot entertain them both at the same time. Choose wisely.

Action Step:

- Quit worrying. Focus on what could go RIGHT.

Self Talk

I'm a big believer in talking to yourself. Yes, sometimes I am worried that I've taken it too far - for instance, when I notice I am talking to myself out loud in public. But, alas, most of the great people of the world seem a little crazy, right? In all seriousness, I talk to myself intentionally. The more difficult a time I am going through, the more I am going to talk to myself. But not just any talking will do; it has to be intentional and focused. I use positive self-talk to shape my mind and attitude, which, in turn, shapes my health and my life.

Whether aloud, or silently in my mind, using my own voice to speak words of power, affirmation, and healing is one of the

best tools for healing that I employ. The words you speak should adhere to the following:
1. Be in the first person.
2. Be in present tense.
3. Be specific.

For example, you might say, "I am healthy, energetic, and at peace in my spirit." One of my long-running favorites was, "I am a healthy, fit, and thin woman, full of inner peace and joy because I make good habits slaves to my burning desire for health, inner peace, and beauty."

Here are some examples of affirmations that are general and easy for anyone to utilize:

I am healthy and vibrant.
I am full of joy and peace.
I am strong and flexible in body, mind, and spirit.
I am focused, energetic, and enthusiastic.
I fill each day with purpose and authenticity.
My body responds to my healthy efforts.
Each day is a new opportunity for finding joy.
I am quick to listen, slow to speak, and easy to forgive.

You don't have to believe the affirmation at first. With enough repetition, you *will* believe it and you will live it! Positive self-talk also doesn't have to be perfectly constructed or memorized. If you are feeling low, simply start speaking words of encouragement to yourself. "I am at peace and full of vitality!" "I love my life and am grateful for my body!" Sometimes, it is as simple as saying, "I'm AWESOME." Simply cut the negative talk and worrying, and replace them with encouraging words that you would give your child or best friend.

Action Step:

- Create a few affirmations that you can read aloud to yourself frequently.
- Post them in two places that you will see them daily.
- Read them to yourself at least three times a day (300 is better!).

Visualization

What you can see in your mind and speak with your tongue, surely you will manifest. On the same lines as speaking is seeing. As a past Child Birth Educator, I was trained both in how to lead guided visualizations, and in the power of them. We tend to manifest what we see in our mind and long for passionately.

For me, I daily take time to visualize myself as I wish to be: full of energy, strong, lean, and balanced. This visualizing is easy to fit in when I wake up in the morning, or am lying down to sleep. It also fits well during my daytime rest periods. It's important to create as much detail as possible in your visualizations. When you visualize yourself, be specific about what you are wearing, what your hair looks like, and where you are. Notice how you feel. These details help to make your visualization real, giving you something tangible to cling to and work toward.

Action Step:

- Daily visualize living and being your healthy, vital self.

Heal Your Spirit

I think that in our modern, civilized lives, we deeply undervalue the state of our spirit. There also seems to be a shift in this area, with more people becoming aware of the need to develop their spiritual life. What I am speaking of here would encompass everything that involves the development of our character, our morals, and our relation to this world via our belief system.

Every one of the major religions teaches moral and character development, and a relationship with the Creator or Divine. Somehow, we "students" have fussed over the details throughout the thousands of years that organized belief systems have been in existence.

As yoga teaches us to create harmony in our body, mind, and spirit, it is with the aim of creating a union with the Divine, or Creator, or God. The teachings of yoga are so strong that they insist we must believe in SOMETHING greater than ourselves, whatever we call it, in order to truly develop in all areas. Do not think the atheist or agnostic is left out in this area. One of my teachers offered this: if you do not believe in a god, or the ability to have a relationship with a god, then cling to the Universe, your Higher Consciousness, or Mother Nature, to give honor and tribute to. The idea is that you must believe in something high and wonderfully powerful.

Faith in something has the ability to lift a soul in a way that nothing else can. By having faith, you have a constant companion,n and a source for prayer and meditation. Faith gives us confidence and power to move through life in a way that minimizes conflict and empowers us in any situation.

Whether you are Muslim, Shaman, Buddhist, Hindu, Christian, Jew, Atheist, Agnostic, or anything else, you have the ability to strengthen your faith and connection with your beliefs. Let yourself become absorbed in the teachings of the prophets, and become more closely aligned with your authentic self by shedding the layers of character that weigh you down.

Action Step:

- Devote time to prayer, meditation, and spiritual development.

In Closing

Action Steps Summary

Getting Started
Action Steps:

- Write a whole page about where you are in life in relation to the ditch and why you are there.
- Make a list of the pros and cons of being right where you are, right now. What are you getting by staying in the ditch (both positive and negative)? What are you missing?
- Then make a list of the pros and cons of healing yourself.
- What will you gain?
- What will you lose?
- Determine your dominant quality of mind.
- List activities and/or foods you can add to your life to bring you toward *sattva*.
- List activities and/or foods you can eliminate from your life to bring you toward *sattva*.
- Make a decision to heal yourself, and write it down. Post it on your refrigerator.
- Create in your mind's eye an image of what a "healthy you" would look and feel like.
- Write down a description of this image/goal.
- Evaluate your schedule and the amount of time you can devote to study.
- Expect to need a minimum of three to six hours a week to do this.

Action Step:

- Identify situations that cause you stress, and choose to either change the situations or change the way you think about them.
- When people get on your nerves, assume the best of them, and don't let them steal your peace.
- Daily, take 10 minutes to be quiet, and breathe deeply. Doing this THREE times a day is optimal. Once a day is a good start.
- You can immediately induce the PNS with a simple exercise. This exercise works every time without fail. Use a yoga block, a thickly-folded blanket, a pillow, or any object you can place beneath your pelvis to elevate your hips 3-5 inches off of a surface you will lie on (if you are obese, stay around 3 inches in elevation). At this height, the exercise is safe for everyone. Some find that the most comfortable option is to place a block on the floor, and lay a folded blanket over the block in a way that it will create a ramp for your back low back. Lie on your back, with this prop under your pelvis, and bending your knees with the soles of your feet on the floor. Place a small, rolled towel under your neck. Rest your arms at your sides, palms up, with enough space between your arms and your body to create space in your arm pits. Take deep, slow breaths. Rest here with your eyes closed for a minimum of 5-10 minutes, twice a day. This will active your PNS immediately, encouraging you to feel more peaceful, and generating your natural energy. Make sure you don't skimp on the time, as it takes four minutes for the PNS to kick in. When you prepare to rise, roll onto your right side, taking a couple of breaths before you gently push yourself up. If you have varicose veins, or simply want

even more benefit from a greater inversion, elevate your feet during this exercise by propping them on a bed, couch, or wall. However, if you have uncontrolled high blood pressure or glaucoma, or are menstruating, don't elevate your feet.
- Go organic
- Filter water
- Filter air
- Replace toiletries and household products with all natural ones
- Cleanse the colon
- Cleanse the liver
- Cleanse the kidneys
- Cleanse the lungs
- Cleanse the skin
- Add infrared sauna to your routine.
- Choose someone to guide you through nutritional supplementation.
- Take your supplements faithfully.
- Get tested for food sensitivities/allergies.
- Get tested for deficiencies and begin supplementation.
- Eliminate offending foods and add healing foods.
- Drink half your body weight in ounces of water a day.
- Build regular rest periods into your schedule, and then take those breaks (even when you don't want to).
- Choose an exercise regimen, set a regular schedule, and stick with it.

Bonus Steps:

- Add Oil Pulling to your routine.
- Add regular massage to your routine.
- Add Ionic Foot Detox to your routine.
- Add essential oils to your routine.

- Add binaural beat and/or classical music to your routine.
- See a chiropractor and/or a Chinese medicine doctor.

Heal Your Mind
Action Step:

- Quit worrying. Focus on what could go RIGHT.
- Create a few affirmations that you can read aloud to yourself frequently.
- Post them in two places that you will see them daily.
- Read them to yourself at least three times a day (300 is better!).
- Daily visualize living and being your healthy, vital self.

Heal Your Spirit
Action Step:

- Devote time to prayer, meditation and spiritual development.

You Can Do It

> *"Our deepest fear is not that we are inadequate. Our deepest fear is that we are powerful beyond measure. It is our light, not our darkness that most frightens us. We ask ourselves, Who am I to be brilliant, gorgeous, talented, fabulous?" Actually, who are you not to be? You are a child of God. Your playing small does not serve the world. There is nothing enlightened about shrinking so that other people won't feel insecure around you. We are all meant to shine, as children do. We were born to make manifest the glory of God that is within us. It's not just in some of us; it's in everyone. And as we let our own light shine, we unconsciously give other people permission to do the same. As we are liberated from our own fear, our presence automatically liberates others."*

Marianne Williamson, "A Return to Love: Reflections on the Principles of 'A Course in Miracles.'" This quote was read by Nelson Mandela at his inaugural speech in 1994.

What I want you to finish this book knowing is that you were designed to be well. You were designed to be healthy, fit, and beautiful, inside and out. The blueprint for you is the same as it was before you were born, and the power to realize it is yours. Through devoted self care, diligent compassion for your efforts, and unending patience, you can heal yourself. You can be more energetic and healthier than you are now, and you can be empowered by the results that you create. Every one of us has 24 hours in a day, and every one of us has the ability to use that time to direct the path of our life. So, stand up, move forward, and be healed!

For most people, it took a long time to become sick and broken, and it could take just as long to reach your goal of health and vitality. When you feel discouraged, ask yourself if it will be worth it to wait that long to be well. What is the alternative? Choosing not to get well doesn't make any sense. So, stick with it, and know that it may not be a fast fix and there are no shortcuts. If you are going to make lasting changes in your body, mind, and spirit, it may take a while, but I can promise you it will be worth it.

###

Thank you for reading my book. It is a first in this topic area, and I hope you found it of benefit. If you enjoyed it, won't you please take a moment to leave me a review at your favorite retailer?

Thanks!

Tara McGuire

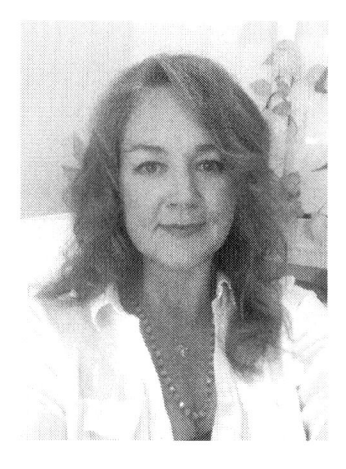

About the Author:

Tara McGuire is an activist and author on the topics of health and healing, pregnancy, birth, personal growth, and empowerment. She has a history as a Certified Childbirth Educator and CCE Trainer through BirthWorks® International, as well as acting as a birth attendant. Currently, Tara is a certified yoga instructor, and co-owns and operates Epídavros Center for Wellbeing and Epídavros Yoga Studio with her husband, Don Marthaller. In addition to these activities, Tara is a home-schooling mother of four children, and surrogate mother to one.

Tara's purpose and mission statement:
The purpose of my life is to experience joy and passion by helping myself and others live life to its highest potential.

Also by Tara McGuire, the book titled:
BIRTH UNHINDERED

Follow me on Facebook: http://facebook.com/taralmcguire

Made in the USA
San Bernardino, CA
04 March 2016